When a meeting is also farewell

COPING WITH A STILLBIRTH OR NEONATAL DEATH

When a meeting is also farewell

COPING WITH A STILLBIRTH OR NEONATAL DEATH

Ingela Rådestad

Translated by David Smith

Books *for* Midwives

Published by Books for Midwives Press
Robert Stevenson House,
1-3 Baxter's Place,
Leith Walk,
Edinburgh EH1 3AF

ISBN 1 898507 75 9

First published 1999
Transferred to digital printing 2003

A catalogue record for this book is available from the British Library.

 your source for books,
journals and multimedia
in the health sciences
www.elsevierhealth.com

For: Ellen

Hedvig

Mårten

Alexander

I have known

you

I can never lose

you

Jacques Werup, *Envoi*, 48 poems from Österlen, Bonniers 1980.

Contents

Foreword

Giving birth to a stillborn baby, or to a baby which dies shortly after birth, is heart-rending and a tragedy. The expectation and joy at the prospect of the new life changes to despair and grief. Often the catastrophe occurs swiftly and unexpectedly, and for the parents, the sudden emotional transformation is devastating. The death of a child also puts a large burden on the staff of a ward where parents and children are cared for.

The thought of writing a book about grieving for a small child came during the summer when I lost my own first child. Ellen died in the womb just a few weeks before the expected birth. It felt important to tell the world about her birth and the boundless grief which followed.

Enduring grief consumes both time and strength. Possibly the period after Ellen's death was unnecessarily difficult. At the hospital we were made to feel unusual because we expressed a desire to be alone for a while with our dead baby. The midwife wiped my hand after I had stroked my baby's cheek. Ellen was not treated with love and care. We were expected to control our feelings, to forget and to look to the future. Even today I feel regret and a loss over the fact that I never was allowed to hold Ellen in my arms.

Five years after Ellen's death I felt able to express something of my feelings related to her death. In the first chapter you can read a modified version of what I wrote then.

What I wrote was published as an article in the journal of the Swedish Midwives Society and received an unexpectedly large response. Many of those who responded had experienced the death of their own children. My correspondence with a colleague, Maria, who lost Alexander three years earlier, can be read in chapter two. The parents of Mårten and Hedvig describe their experiences in the following chapters.

The discussions with those who responded to the article indicated the need for a book on the subject, and that there was not much written for those parents who had suffered such a loss.

My hope is that this book will be used in the basic and advanced education and training of doctors, midwives, nurses, nursing auxiliaries, medical social workers and psychologists. My message to you is simple: Take part in the parents' time together with the baby. This is a farewell, help it to be a moving and lasting memory. It may seem remarkable that the birth of a stillborn child or a child which soon dies need not only be tragic. My belief is that you will understand what I mean when you have read our accounts in this book.

I also believe that your professional efforts on such occasions can give much satisfaction. Meta, who is a midwife on a maternity ward, describes more in the chapter 'Be close, listen and be there...'.

The book has also been written for you, if you have lost a baby. Possibly this has happened recently? Then this can be a difficult subject to read about, memories are brought back to life, you may cry. Cry freely, your baby is worth crying over. It is a difficult time.

My hope is that our book will help to break the isolation one can feel as a parent who has suffered such a loss. Hopefully we will be able to convey a belief in the future and show you that out of your grief can grow aspects of life of which you were not previously aware. The day will almost certainly come when even you will agree with Birgitta's words spoken in the book: 'I have been given a valuable experience, one which I would have preferred to be without and instead been allowed to keep Hedvig'. When one has suffered such a loss and felt such grief it is possible to go back out into the world a stronger person. Maria wrote in a letter: 'The day we buried Alexander, when all that we wished for was to feel his heartbeat, I believed that we never again could be happy. Never properly happy. I am not so certain now. It is true that I cry more easily than before Alexander's death but I also feel that I shall find it easier to laugh'.

Finally I would like to thank all of you who have helped bring this book to fruition. It has meant a lot to me to share your experiences as well as sensing your willingness to relate so openly. Thank you all who have commmented on the manuscript and encouraged me to continue. Without your help there would not have been a book.

Foreword to the English Edition

When the first edition of this book was published in Sweden it filled a void for parents who had lost a baby to neonatal death, as well being useful for medical staff. I have received many letters and had many telephone conversations which bear witness as to how these personal accounts have helped at a difficult time. Today in Sweden, the book is used on medical courses and is given by hospitals to those who have lost a baby at birth. When I started to write the book it was to try to understand my own grief and why I felt as I did. By listening to others who had lost a baby, I could better reach my own feelings. Today Ellen's birth feels distant but she is still there, a sadness, a gentle, veiled grief. I have given birth to three children after Ellen; Isabell, Nils and Martina. They are all well and healthy. My family is such a blessing, but there will always be one child missing.

The need for more understanding of how the health service can best support parents who have lost a baby has led to my undertaking, in recent years, a research project. My thesis concerns women's experience of losing a baby before its birth and also describes how postnatal care influences a woman's welfare several years after the baby's stillbirth. In the last chapter of this book I have included some of the project's results, these do not constitute part of the Swedish edition of the book. I am now Ph.D., Dr.Med.Sc. and work as a senior lecturer at the Department of Caring Sciences at Mälardalens University in Sweden.

Health care during pregnancy and labour can vary between countries, and even within a country. Some of the routines described in the book may not be relevant in the British Isles. In Sweden the midwife carries out normal antenatal care as well as normal deliveries. Where an intra-uterine death occurs, it is not uncommon for the midwife to become an especially significant person.

Many have contributed to this book. Let me thank David Smith who made this translation so sensitive to the original. Also, I am indebted to my husband Gunnar Steineck for editorial suggestions.

Ingela Rådestad

Introduction

Sweden has a population of under nine million and there are approximately 100 000 births each year. The country has a very low rate of intrauterine and perinatal death but even so about 700 such deaths occur annually.

On average a woman makes 10 visits to her antenatal clinic with a booking appointment normally taking place between the twelfth and fourteenth weeks of pregnancy. There is currently a trend away from routine care to a system where resources are directed to those cases requiring a greater degree of care.

The overall aim is for antenatal care to provide complete medical supervision during pregnancy. Complications cannot be eliminated, but with regular and properly conducted examinations and tests any potential injury may be reduced through early action. Where required, some social support is also provided by the midwife.

Medical supervision is intended to:

– identify specific factors which increase the risk for complications

- eliminate the cause of illness or make the patient the subject of special supervision

- identify illnesses and complications where optimally applied resources may reduce or eliminate any injury to the mother or child.

Antenatal care and the available facilities can vary from clinic to clinic. A pregnant woman does have some choice regarding delivery unit and method for the birth. A programme is prepared for each mother-to-be. The aim of the programme is to facilitate the identification of any irregularities in the development or growth of the fetus as well as any illness or condition of the mother which may be significant for the pregnancy, the birth or the development of the fetus.

The mother-to-be will normally see a doctor at a second visit which takes place shortly after the first. At subsequent visits she will expect generally to see the same midwife. 99% of mothers have at least one ultrasound scan and this is usually carried out during the seventeenth week of pregnancy. Nearing term the pregnant woman will visit her midwife more frequently.

Most clinics can provide antenatal courses for all of their expectant parents. Groups of six or seven couples meet for about two hours on about six occasions. Virtually 100% of primigravida participate whereas only about 20% of multigravida participate in the courses.

Where there are no anticipated complications the delivery is managed by a midwife. A doctor takes over responsibility where the delivery is complicated or a Caesarean section is necessary. During the nineties approximately 10-15% of babies have been delivered by Caesarean section. After the birth most women stay in hospital for two or three days but some choose to return home more or less immediately.

Antenatal care, the delivery and postnatal care in Sweden are free. There are several types of benefit applicable in connection with pregnancy and the birth of a child. Sickness benefit is available and results normally in a relatively small shortfall in income. Where a woman is obliged to reduce her working hours she is entitled to a percentage of benefit relative to the reduction in hours worked. A woman who has a physically demanding job or works in an environment which may cause injury to the fetus, may receive benefit if alternative working conditions cannot be arranged.

Parental benefit is available for up to 15 months and may be shared between the parents. This benefit can be utilised until the child is eight years old. For the mother's part this benefit is available before the birth but no earlier than 60 days before term. The father, within a period of 60 days after the birth, is entitled to 10 days paternity leave.

Swedish definitions

Perinatal death:

- A child which is stillborn after the end of the 28th week of pregnancy.
- Where the length of the pregnancy is uncertain: a child which is stillborn and is at least 35cm long.
- A child which is born alive but which dies within seven days of the birth.

British definitions

Perinatal death: a baby which dies during the first week of life.

Neonatal death: an infant which dies within one month of its birth.

Stillbirth: A baby, born after the 24th completed week of pregnancy, which does not breathe or show other signs of life after being expelled from the body of its mother.

Some children who suffer perinatal death have defects which prevent them from surviving outside the womb. Complications related to the placenta and umbilical cord can cause stillbirth. Other children are premature and die, for example, because their lungs do not function properly

4

or because they have a severe infection. Some parents receive no explanation as to why their baby has died.

Sweden has one of the lowest rates of child mortality in connection with delivery. Today, approximately 5 out of 1000 children suffer a perinatal death; of these just over half are stillborn.

In 1994 the perinatal death rate in Sweden was 5.4 per 1000 births. In the United Kingdom the corresponding figure was 8.9 and in the United States it was 7.9. In 1996, 5.2 perinatal deaths per 1000 births were registered in Sweden, and 8.7 per 1000 births in the United Kingdom. Figures from the OECD Health Database comprise early neonatal deaths (deaths under seven days) plus deaths of 28 weeks of gestation or more, per 1000 total births.

To meet and part in the same instant

Here is the story of how Ellen was born.

I was one of 380 women who that year, according to official Swedish statistics, gave birth to a stillborn child.

I was working full-time as a nurse on a surgical ward. At the same time I was expecting my first child. I felt fit and well, and I had a tan from the winter sun. My pregnancy was normal, all test results were satisfactory and it was hinted that it was almost unnecessary to carry out antenatal checks on someone as healthy as I was. My visits to the clinic were therefore cut to every third week instead of every second week which, is normal towards the end of a pregnancy.

It was during a visit to the midwife, the Thursday in my thirty fifth week, that my blood pressure was found to be high. 'Nothing to worry about', said the midwife.

My urine contained some protein. 'Three plusses but it's probably just a touch of cystitis', was the comforting comment.

The next day I gave a sample for an Esbach's test, to measure the level of protein. After a busy day at work in the hospital I went back to the antenatal clinic to be told the result.

'Two grams, that's slightly too much', said the midwife. A doctor came in and, standing in the doorway, signed a sick-note. 'A sick-note, why? How can one feel so healthy and yet be given a sick-note?' I asked. The doctor talked to me about pre-eclampsia. He assumed that I was acquainted with the illness because I was a nurse.

'Take it easy over the weekend. You'll be well looked after at home', said the doctor, referring to the fact that my husband worked on the hospital's medical ward as a doctor. I didn't get round to mentioning the fact that my husband would be away for the weekend.

I dutifully took things easy and had a bad conscience for having made things difficult and for being ill. Now the new nurse on my ward would not get a proper introduction. I also started to read my husband's books, especially the sections about cramp due to pre-eclampsia and about how pregnant women can die. For the first time I became frightened. My stomach felt strange, at times the womb became hard. I remember thinking that it was the baby turning. I had been told that the baby would move less now that the head was in position and the fact that I did not feel any movement was, I thought, normal. At the same time that my fears became greater, I tried to convince myself that everything would be fine at my next appointment on Monday.

The Result

At long last, Monday morning! It is a relief to go to the clinic with all my questions which have been forming during the weekend. My blood pressure is slightly up on Friday's level and my urine contains the same amount of protein. 'The rest has not done a lot of good', I think to myself. The midwife takes the fetal stethoscope to listen to the baby's heartbeat. She cannot find it and searches at different places on my stomach. It is unpleasant and the womb becomes hard. The midwife has a serious and resolute look. I am not feeling worried as she has not been close to the point where the heartbeat was counted last time. Now she is placing the fetal stethoscope at exactly the same place as last Thursday and she holds it there a long while. 'Why is she not looking at her watch while counting the heartbeats?' I wonder. The midwife removes the fetal stethoscope saying something about it being difficult to to hear the heartbeat. She says that she is going to telephone the labour ward where the heartbeat can be registered using CTG, a method which is more sensitive and reliable than using a fetal stethoscope. My silent dialogue begins. 'If they are going to use CTG there must be a heartbeat. If there isn't a heartbeat then they can't run a CTG trace, therefore there is a heartbeat and the baby must be alive.'

On the labour ward the wait seems endless before an assistant comes to take me to the machine. I observe her movements and see that she has done this many times before. She chats all the while. 'How long before you are due to give birth? Is it a boy or girl?' she asks. I answer simply, because I cannot concentrate on anything but the trace and the search for the heartbeat. The assistant is busy with the CTG-machine.

'How strange', she says as she twists the dials. She moves the probe around on my stomach which is sticky with contact gel. She turns pale and her cordiality disappears, she is mumbling instead of talking. Suddenly she leaves the room.

'I'm just going to fetch a midwife', she says. The door closes behind her. I wait. The midwife comes in and tries to obtain contact between the baby and the machine. Even she gives up after a while without getting anywhere. She looks me in the eye, a look of pity and understanding. I know that she knows, that which I have already begun to realise: the baby is not alive any more.

'It doesn't look good', says the midwife. A doctor is called.

'Ultrasound is a more reliable means of checking the heart's activity', says the midwife to me. 'Of course,' I think, 'ultrasound will show the heart's beat'. It could be so clearly seen in the seventeenth week of my pregnancy and I remember the feeling of pride when I saw my child for the first time on the ultrasound screen.

The specialist arrives, it is his first day at the clinic. He says his name indistinctly, not once looking me in the eye during his examination. The specialist is talking about me to the midwife. No heartbeat is discernible. I wonder if it is not necessary to X-ray my stomach to see if the baby has died. I can see that they think that it is an unnecessary examination. Even so, the doctor writes out an X-ray request form, possibly to avoid having to tell me that the baby is dead.

I have to wait for a long time at the X-ray department. A student nurse, working extra as an assistant, comes in to keep me company. She seeks contact in an obtrusive way; I see that she thinks of me as an interesting case. In her eagerness to discover as much as possible, possibly to tell her class colleagues later on, she is totally devoid of feeling for my situation.

'How old are you?' asks the student nurse. 'Imagine that, you're the same age as I am', she says when I have answered. 'To think that you're a nurse, the same as I am going to be.'

'Leave me alone', I am thinking at the same time as I am answering her questions. I do not have the energy to ask her to go.

The X-ray shows nothing more than the ultrasound already has. When I am told the result at the X-ray department, the student nurse is still with me. The tears start to flow. Not violently, I am just quietly weeping for myself.

'At least you're crying', says the student, as if she has just discovered that I have feelings.

Back on the labour ward, practical details are discussed. I am to be admitted to a gynaecological ward and induced the day after. I may stay at the hospital if I wish, but I choose to meet my husband who is arriving by plane in a few hours. Telling him is going to be the hardest part – four days earlier he left behind joy and optimism and now he is coming home to this tragedy. A paralyzing cramp hits us as we share the knowledge. We go home, lie down on the bed which is transformed into a raft on a malevolent sea. In the afternoon I am admitted to the ward and a new ultrasound examination is carried out by the regular doctor. This time there is a dialogue between the examiner and ourselves. Mostly we discuss what is going to take place and why the baby has died.

The birth

My husband and I are allowed to share a room overnight. The next morning we go back to the labour ward at half past nine. The midwife, older and experienced, misses three times when trying to insert the needle for the drip. She becomes irritated and finally seeks help from an anaesthetics nurse. I have been promised as much anaesthesia as I require. A local anaesthetic round the cervix is to be administered as soon as possible. The regular doctor is to be on hand throughout the whole delivery. We feel great confidence in him.

'How quickly should the drip be administered?', we wonder.

'Seeing that there isn't a baby to consider, there's no need to take things slowly', says the midwife. She sets the drip at 10 drops per minute and quickly increases the rate to 15. My womb reacts violently to the hormones in the fluid. The contractions are continuous and it hurts. My husband becomes worried when my blood pressure rises. I am given a pain-killing injection. The contractions are very strong. The midwife does not look to see how much the cervix has dilated, despite the fact that we ask her to.

'You've only had the drip for an hour, and this can take all day', she says. When my blood pressure has risen even further my husband becomes yet more worried. I notice that the midwife is annoyed with him, thinking that he is involving himself too much. Even so, she rings the doctor and is given permission to administer anti-hypertensive drugs, to reduce my blood pressure.

I begin to feel a lot of pain and there is no pause between the contractions. When the midwife wishes to increase the drip rate even further my husband asks if it is not possible to lower it instead so that I may rest for a while.

'Rest? We must get this over and done with', says the midwife, with a displeased glance at my husband. She notices, however, that I am in a lot of pain and mumbles that it possibly is about time for more pain relief. The doctor is called and is quickly on the scene. He prepares the anaesthetic and during the examination sees that my cervix is almost fully dilated. He injects as much anaesthetic as possible and we are quickly moved to the delivery suite.

At half past eleven on Tuesday our daughter is born. She is small, has dark hair and we think that she is very beautiful. My husband is standing next to me, holding my head in his hands. We lean forward to see her the moment she is delivered. Our tears flow together.

We ask to be alone together with our daughter for a few moments. The midwife comes in with her on a plastic tray, covered with a sheet. She does not leave the room. I want to hold my baby but I dare not. I caress my daughter's cheek but at the same time I am frightened. The whole time I am aware of my midwife's disapproval; her back as she pretends to clean the hand-basin in the room, at the same time glancing at what we are doing. My husband counts our baby's fingers and toes, we are pleased that she is well formed and beautiful. When the midwife takes our daughter away, she wipes my hand with a cloth soaked in disinfectant. Our feeling of having done something wrong is reinforced.

A lot later I hear that the midwife thought that we were strange for having touched the dead child. She had talked to a colleague and said that we might catch something from the baby. Indignantly, she referred to Semmelweiss, the Hungarian physician who proved that puerperal fever is contagious.

The time after

After the birth came a long period of grief. We met people, both within the health service and friends, who supported us and were very understanding. This is being written five years later. I have given birth to two children who are alive and are healthy. I am now myself a qualified midwife and have often asked myself the question, 'Why did we not receive respect and understanding at Ellen's birth?'. We were not allowed to feel fondness for our daughter, and that has made grieving as well as everything else a lot harder. Probably these past five years would have been very different if we had been allowed to be alone with our daughter.

It is a tragedy to give birth to a stillborn child; however the birth of a stillborn child is, just like the birth of a living child, a powerful, vital, shared experience for the parents. Now, a lot later, when I feel able to summarize my impressions of my first child's birth, this is my most important message: Do not destroy the positive aspects for the parents. It is a child which has been born, a creation of the parents even if it is dead. Each child, even if it is dead and deformed, is thought of as a miracle. They have the right to love their child. The birth is the parents' meeting with the child, a meeting which is also farewell. The meeting can, despite the pain, be a precious and lasting memory which makes it easier to continue life without the awaited child.

Letters from Maria

17 November

Hello Ingela,

I was touched by your story in the magazine 'Jordemodern', and I broke into a cold sweat. I decided to write to you and try to describe what happened in my case.

In January, almost three years ago, my husband and I were expecting our second child. During my pregnancy I trained to be a midwife and, once qualified, I worked for a few months on a labour ward. I had only assisted at ordinary births, with screaming babies which I laid on their mothers' stomachs. I started my maternity leave shortly before Christmas. New Year was celebrated with my parents in my home town.

On New Year's Day, after going to the pictures, I notice that my usually lively baby has not moved for some time. It is quite still in my large stomach. Hours pass with growing unease. At midnight we go to the nearest hospital. I have already telephoned and told them of our fears.

We are met by the same midwife to whom I had spoken on the telephone. She shows my husband to a waiting room. He does not want to leave me, asks stubbornly to be allowed to follow me into the examination room and almost has to force his way in to be with me. The midwife asks me about contractions and the waters and speculates about our making it to our own hospital at home. I repeat what I have said to her on the telephone; that I just want to know if it is possible to hear the baby's heartbeat and that I am worried about how the baby is.

The midwife takes a fetal stethoscope and begins to search for a heartbeat. The room is silent. After a while the midwife breaks the silence by saying that she is going to fetch a CTG-machine. When she returns she places the probe on my stomach, at a spot where I do not think that there is a chance of registering a heartbeat. Suddenly, she says that the machine is probably broken, that they have a lot to do on the ward tonight, and that she will telephone the doctor. When she is on her way out of the room I ask her if she had heard a heartbeat.

'Yes I think so... there...', says the midwife, pointing at my stomach as she leaves the room.

The doctor arrives to carry out an ultrasound examination. He sits with his back towards me and his eyes on the machine. After a while he says aloud, as if to himself, 'It's dead!'. I look up at the machine's screen, seeing the eternally etched picture: The heart, its location, where nothing is moving. My husband and I start to cry, my husband bellows out his pain. The doctor, undisturbed, continues to move the probe around on my stomach. He tells us that we can do as we like, stay or go to the hospital at home. 'There's nothing we can do', he says.

We choose to stay awhile at the hospital; it feels impossible to manage the journey home. My husband and I are shown to a room and the door is closed behind us. Nobody comes in. We feel that we must get out, there's nobody here who wants to have anything to do with us! We dress and start to leave. All of a sudden the midwife is stung into action. She has plenty to say now; we have to take with us a form which shows that we have visited the clinic. We came with a baby and we leave with a piece of paper. The time is half past one. It has never been so cold and so dark, we are completely alone.

The next morning we journey home and then to the labour ward which is also where I work. Everything feels completely empty. I am unable to string two thoughts together, everything happens automatically. People talk to us, touch us. I am crying, my husband's teeth are clenched. After a few hours the birth is induced. Now I know that what I have been waiting for, for such a long time, is going to happen, I shall give birth and I have been looking forward to it.

We have a wonderful midwife and we talk a lot to her. Her greatest attribute is that she helps me to understand that it is a child we are having. Not a dead monster, not a fetus, but a child. A local anaesthetic is placed round the cervix, but I do not wish to have complete pain relief, thinking that it is better to feel the pain. It is as if the physical pain relieves the mental pain.

I can feel the contractions, things happen quickly. The baby arrives before the cervix is fully dilated, or it comes at the same time. It hurts. Someone squeezes my hand, my face is wet from my husband's tears. The midwife is crying. I can feel when the baby's body leaves mine and, although I inwardly expected him to scream, there is a silence. My husband tells me that we have another boy. 'Give him to me', I say, and he is quickly placed in my arms.

We place warm blankets around him. We touch him, caress him, he is unbelievably beautiful. We give him a name. While I am being stitched, and my vulva swabbed, my husband holds the baby. They are standing, alone together, by the window. After a while we are left to ourselves with our son. We place him in a small bed wrapped in his blankets while we drink a cup of coffee. The midwife looks in now and then, but for the most part it is just we two. We have two hours, two hours which should have been a lifetime. The midwife comes in and says that she wishes to take him. Now I know that a heart can break, because mine does. I do not know how I shall be able to let him go, to be taken from me. Even now, whilst writing this, the tears start to flow. My heart starts to break a little again.

Before I am discharged I see my child a second time, I need to hold him in my arms again. My husband brings a camera. We are allowed to be alone in a room where someone has lit a candle. It is lovely and it does not matter that our son has changed colour. It feels good to hold him again. Possibly it is not quite as difficult to be separated from him this time. His cold body tells us that it is necessary. I still feel a little upset that it was then that we photographed him and not when he was newly born. Alexander newly born is the memory which I would prefer to retain.

What passes for postnatal care suddenly stops. Our appointment, to which we have looked forward, turns out to be little more than a statement that they have not found a reason for the baby's death, a gynaecological examination and then we are home again. Nobody from the hospital contacts us. We suffer great personal crises which reach a climax after six months. Someone tells me that divorce is a common result of an experience such as ours and I become powerlessly angry. What is the use of having statistics if nobody makes use of them? Why were we left to our own devices when the risk that we would separate was so great? It did not happen, but it has taken a lot of time and a lot of therapy before things have returned to normal. I believe that we suffered more than was necessary.

Now, almost three years later, I have an insight which is difficult to convey. My third child, born in the summer, is asleep in its cot: a girl a lot like her brother. We have a grave. Our dead son has his place in our family even if physically it is always empty.

There are a lot of things that one would wish to be self-evident in such a situation. Information should be given in a prudent manner, so that it does not lead people closer to the abyss. There may only be one message but there is more than one way to say it. The pain that we, the staff, feel is only a fraction of what the parents are suffering on such occasions.

A chance for the parents to be alone, for as long as they wish, with the baby ought to be available. The process one must always go through before being ready for separation from one's child must happen in a time-span which has been very much shortened, but the process must be allowed to take time; one accepts the need to release the child when the time feels right. It is the parents who should decide when that should take place, not the staff.

There must be the opportunity for one to say to the child all that one wishes, and to create a lasting memory. This one occasion can never be repeated, can never be redone. Our two hours with Alexander still feels too short. If anyone had tried to deny us our son, I would have fought. It was a very strong emotion.

This subject was never taken up during my midwifery training. We received only a handout, a bitter pill after my own experience. It is difficult to be a midwife on such an occasion. All aspects of grief are not pleasant. But all aspects must be allowed to surface if one is to be a complete person afterwards.

I shall now finish this letter which has been waiting to be written for a long time. I shall put to one side your wonderful article, it feels like a bond between sisters.

Sincerely,
Maria

Maria,

Thank you for your wonderful letter, I was deeply moved. It all seemed so familiar when you describe how you were told that Alexander was dead. To be looked upon as an object and not as a person. Meeting a doctor who makes a diagnosis but does not take responsibility for the feelings that are unleashed. I am reminded of how helpless one is and how dependent, in such circumstances, on other people.

I did not have the same strength of character as you did during the birth, to ask to be allowed to hold my baby in my arms. Even if I had asked, I am not at all certain that the midwife would have allowed me to. I am convinced that I would feel much better now if I had been able to hold my daughter in my arms. When one has carried a baby in the womb for several months and become accustomed to feeling it there inside one, the whole of one's being demands to be able to hold the baby, to protect it and give it love.

When our second child was born, just less than a year after Ellen died, she was very poorly and was placed in an incubator. Isabell, as we have called her, was born a month early and her lungs were not fully developed. I remember how strong my feeling was that I was going to hold this child in my arms, come what may. Even today I feel sorrow at the thought of the contact with my first baby which I was denied. I was never given the opportunity to show my love for Ellen. This probably sounds a bit strange to those who have not gone through such an experience but I believe that you understand what I mean.

You wrote, 'What passes for postnatal care suddenly stops'. I can only agree with you. My check-up was, like yours, a simple physical examination. The doctor did not ask how I felt inside. It was summer when Ellen was born. My husband and I went away after the short funeral which took place at the cemetery. We talked a lot to each other and I did think that, after our summer together, I had got over it all. I longed for a baby and felt ready for a new pregnancy.

Coming home was difficult. I felt people's gaze was drawn to the place where my swollen stomach had been, as if to get confirmation of the fact that our baby had died. I quickly became pregnant again and believed that everything would be back to normal as soon as I had the new baby. Now, much later, I realise that it was all too soon. The new pregnancy was difficult with several complications. My grief for Ellen had to take a back seat.

We moved when our second child was a few weeks old. It was a pleasure to leave the small community where it felt as though we were branded as 'those who lost the baby'. We were anonymous in our new home town. We were 'the happy new family'. Nobody knew what had gone before. At the same time it was very frustrating not knowing how to answer when anyone asked how many children I had, if Isabell had any brothers or sisters. I felt as though I was lying when I replied that I only had one daughter. I had various symptoms, racing heart, a cold sweat, dizziness and feeling sick, I thought that I was seriously ill.

It was not until Nils' birth a year ago that I started to admit Ellen's existence to myself and to others. I read several articles in magazines which dealt with the loss of very small children. I discovered reactions to grief described in such a way that I was able to recognise my own. Perhaps there was nothing wrong with me after all. I read about how important it is for parents to see and to hold their dead child, for memories to be formed.

I was encouraged to write the article about my own experience of losing a baby after I met a mother on the ward where I was working. A few days before, she had given birth to a daughter and, as far as I could see, she was filled with anguish. She was tense, troubled and her breastfeeding was not going well. On reading her medical notes I saw that two years earlier she had given birth to a stillborn baby. I asked her if we could talk about her first child, at the same time telling her about my own baby which had died. We talked for a long time about her baby, her grief and the difficulties with the new baby.

Afterwards the mother was transformed, she was calmer, more relaxed and happy. Breastfeeding started to function and shortly afterwards she left the maternity unit. With my article I wished to try to convey to our colleagues how important the midwife is to parents who lose a baby.

I would like to thank you for your wonderful letter, please get in touch if it feels right.

Warm greetings,
Ingela

Ingela,

Your letter filled our Saturday with thoughts. It developed
into a late night. It was a reason for us to talk about that
which we now rarely discuss. I have never previously
exchanged thoughts with someone who has gone through
the same thing.

I recognise so well my own experience. I have been caused
much heart-searching by the question of how many
children I have. If I said, 'One child', it felt like treason.
If I answered, 'Two', and tried to explain, the person
who had asked gave me a strange look and that also made
me feel uncomfortable. Sometimes I feel like being
provocative and protesting against the custom which
forces us to keep a 'stiff upper lip'. Now I normally
answer, 'I have given birth to three children but we lost
one'. That generally is sufficient.

If the midwife at the birth had not reinforced the feeling
within me that I was the mother of two children, and if
I had not had the opportunity to have Alexander with
me, I do not think that I would be able to say it as naturally
as I can today.

A short time after Alexander's birth I read an article
about children who die at birth. Amongst other things it
said that it is common for a woman to feel herself to be
a failure if she loses her baby. I thought about this and tried

to search my own feelings. No, that was not the way I felt. A lot later, about half a year, the article's message was confirmed for me. The fiasco hit me full in the face. I felt disapproval, rejected by life. A failure. It did not make any difference that I had earlier given birth to a living, healthy, bouncing baby. That could have been luck.

It caused me a lot of pain and it was not something that I could talk about. There was a feeling of extreme loneliness. Unfortunately I had started work again on the labour ward where Alexander was born. It was not a fortunate combination and probably the reason why my 'career' as midwife has never felt quite right. Delivering other women's babies was a daily rape of myself. With each baby I delivered, my own sense of fiasco grew. I really begrudged others their babies. It was a bitter, undisguised jealousy. I hated pregnant women, not to mention the babies. After a few months I admitted to myself that this was the case and I allowed myself to have these feelings despite the fact that it required quite an effort. I started working as a night nurse on a surgical ward and that was a relief.

What took even longer, and was infinitely more difficult to admit to myself, was that I was insanely angry at Alexander. You know, when one starts to kick at stones when out taking a walk. One is angry without knowing the reason. Eventually I could say to him, 'You let me down, you didn't approve of me and I despise you'.

Days pass by. I need a break from my thoughts and feelings. The realisation that one does not only have positive thoughts about a defenceless person, a baby – it is still a shameful thing to talk about. I have heard from midwives that this reaction can even come during the birth. I feel sorry for these parents. Not because of their feelings but because I believe that they cause a negative reaction amongst the staff. Despair can be accepted, but aggression? To be allowed to hate Alexander was necessary, in order to be able once again to love him. It was just so impossible, so unacceptable to have such feelings.

In general I have experienced so much after Alexander's death that life has become richer. I thought that I understood people who dyed their hair green, understood what they felt and cried out for. I wanted to protest against this injustice in life which had taken Alexander from me. I was too 'grown-up' to dye my hair green but I felt the same things. It was a crossroads in my life. The event has formed a clear boundary between the old and the new me, and possibly between me and many other people.

I think of how wrong it can all turn out, depending on how we the staff think of our own role and significance. If we underrate this then we become like the doctor who carried out the ultrasound scan on me. Perhaps he was thinking, 'This situation is so awful that it doesn't matter what I say. Therefore I won't take any responsibility for this. I'll carry out this ultrasound scan and ascertain that the baby is dead. Whatever I say, or don't say, will be irrelevant.'

If we overrate our significance we can easily seize up. For example, reasoning along these lines: 'I have to be able to say something which helps these people. I don't know what to say but I have to say something.' And it becomes so incredibly important to have something sensible to say that one does not discover one's own feelings of sympathy or understanding.

So many strange things have happened around us. One of the most remarkable was that we soon felt required to exhibit common-sense. Nobody made any allowances when we said odd things, nobody could understand. It seemed as though the world consisted of people who went about not giving the game away, and who were sensible and clever. Surely we could not be the only ones feeling grief? We were defenceless. It was something which I thought would get better with time but I am much more vulnerable today than I was before.

My husband has had to learn to cope with his role as a man. Men have definitely not to show their feelings. He was off work for two weeks after Alexander's death but that was for my sake. My husband never felt that he counted, neither at the hospital nor later.

We have been left to go through the different phases of reaction to a crisis, phases which I have grown to distrust and dislike. It is easy to put a label on things if one does not scratch the surface. A long, long time I waited to go through the phase of acceptance, feeling the mockery. To be given a sick-note for 'psychological insufficiency', what does it mean really? To be in a world where everyone is striving not to show their feelings, whilst one has, oneself, the ability to react: what, then, is insufficiency?

I know that December will soon become January. Soon it will be Alexander's third birthday. Time does change one's perspective. Often Alexander seems diffuse, gone; at other times it is as if he is right here, as though I am once again holding him in my arms. It feels as though something threatening is approaching, even though I know today that it does not need lead to a crisis. But a gentle memory, can that be anything to hope for?

Friendly greetings,
Maria

19 January

Maria,

Alexander's birthday, how did it go? It is often written in literature that birthdays can be difficult occasions, even many years after a child's death. It has been different for me. Ellen's first birthday was pushed into the background by our second child who was then nine days old. I was completely consumed by my role as a new mother. I realise now that it was entirely wrong that the new baby pushed Ellen to one side in that way. I pushed my unfinished grieving away. Even her other birthdays have passed without reflection. It has taken until the latest, the fifth birthday, for a change to come about. It took five years for me to be able to accept my first child.

On her fifth birthday we went to the town where Ellen was born and took with us a large armful of white carnations, the same flowers as we had at her funeral. We know where she is buried but the grave is unmarked, there is no stone with her name on it. I regret it now, that we do not have a grave just for her. We told the children about their older sister. For me it was a wonderful birthday. Obviously it was tinged with some sorrow but mostly I felt myself to be in harmony. Psycholgical balance brought on by the realisation that I have come to terms with my feelings for my first child. To admit to myself that Ellen did exist. We even visited the hospital where Ellen and Isabell were born. For me it was important to see the

33

room where she was born, to look in the delivery book and to see the red cross next to Ellen's identity number.

Maria, you wrote in your first letter that you went through a crisis half a year after Alexander's death. How did you find help to get through the crisis?

You write of your anger. When I was a student midwife I met a woman who had just given birth to her second child. A few years earlier her first child had died at birth. When she talked about what had happened it was with a fury directed towards the doctor who she thought was responsible for her baby's death. She never expressed any sadness for her loss and I got the impression that she found it difficult to be pleased at the arrival of her new baby. It would seem that it is important to express our anger, and not get embroiled in it.

Your letter reminded me of my own anger, a feeling I had almost entirely suppressed. It was directed towards the mothers in the nursery on the other side of the corridor. They stood, bent over the cots, smiling and babbling with their new-born babies. I used to think, 'What have you done to deserve having a healthy, living child?'. Life was so unfair! If I saw a pregnant woman or a new mother smoking, things felt even harder. They should have given birth to a stillborn child instead of me. I had at least done my best during my pregnancy and those who were smoking were surely not worthy of having a baby.

I remember a trip to the south of Sweden after Ellen's death. We stopped at several beaches. Parents were there with their children. My husband and I commented on the parents' unsuitable psychological contact with their children. What poor parents we thought that they were, and how good we would have been if our child had been allowed to live. I could not bear to hear someone complaining over how demanding their children were. One should be thankful for the great joy of having a living child.

You write of the phases of a reaction to a crisis. A woman told me that after her child's death, the nurse who talked to her stood there with a book about reactions to crises in her hand. She was trying to work out where the mother was in her passage through the crisis, and from time to time quoted passages from the book. This must surely be a misunderstanding of the models of grief which have been formulated. At the same time I think that it was a shortcoming that nobody told us that it was important to release those feelings that grief wakens, and that it takes a long time to regain one's balance or achieve stability. We were encouraged to keep our courage up and be strong. I now realise that it takes a lot of work to come through a loss like this if one hopes to emerge unharmed. Five years ago I thought that grief would only last a few months. Today I have an entirely different perspective concerning the time required.

Warmly,
Ingela

Ingela,

The summer after Alexander's birth was difficult. I telephoned different hospitals and therapists seeking help to take us out of the crisis. Everywhere was closed for the holidays. In desperation I turned to a medical social worker at the gynaecological clinic, we had met her once earlier and talked about the funeral. The social worker provisionally arranged a meeting with a counsellor at the children's psychiatric unit. This could be managed because we already had a child. An express train went through our home, a ball started rolling at great speed. There was a considerable distance between my husband and myself. We met the counsellor four times and she tried to help us listen to each other. Then she went on holiday and I continued with another counsellor.

We had sessions each week during the autumn. It required a lot of effort. The discussions did not so much concern Alexander but more the relationship between my husband and myself and everything that had been brought to the surface by our deep sorrow. The therapy sessions finished around Christmas. In retrospect, that was a bit too soon. The first anniversary and the time around it was very difficult. At that time I thought that I would never be free from that wild grief. About the time of the anniversary my husband sought help and started therapy sessions which continued for a year. They have given him a lot of support.

The third anniversary went quite well. I felt a lump in my throat all day. But it was only for that day. It is so easy to recall the memory of my pregnancy, but on this occasion I actually avoided getting close to it.

We have a fine grave in a cemetery situated in the woods. A stone marked with his name stands in a glade. I often go there, but on Alexander's birthdays I am not able to make myself go. I make plans to go there and light a candle, but when the day comes I just cannot. It is strange because I can go there on any other day. But on the birthdays I need all my strength just to survive.

Peter, Alexander's elder brother, sometimes asks how old his little brother is. It has been a great help to see at close quarters how a child handles disappointment and thoughts of death. In the beginning it was, despite everything, important for him to be a big brother. We stressed this and gave him support but the shine wore off when the brother or sister did not arrive. Peter soon learned that it was possible for him to laugh even though I was crying. I have noticed that in recent years he has stopped asking why I am crying. My crying does not seem to affect him noticeably. A year ago we read 'Brothers Lionheart' by Astrid Lindgren. Despite the fact that we have never talked about it, Peter said spontaneously, 'Alexander's in Nangijala now. How old is he there? Imagine being able to ride a horse when you are only three!' For Peter it is natural that Alexander lives in Nangijala and that we are here.

Peter often tells his younger sister that we have another child: 'You may also get a little brother who dies'. I remember the open grief in his face the day that, full of expectation, he came to me in the hospital. Peter cried, asked why and talked about other babies which did not die.

We talk at times about Alexander who should be here, we all feel this strongly. That was the way things were when Lina was born. She came to all the family, to two older brothers. By accepting Peter's view, life has become easier and I even learn things from him. Peter will be seven this summer and I think that he is wonderfully sensible. He will be back from nursery school in five minutes so I shall finish now.

Many greetings,
Maria

Maria and I continued to write to each other during the Spring. We met in May and I told Maria about my interviews with other parents who have borne a loss and about my idea for a book. On the second of July, Maria wrote a concluding letter, intended for this book. Maria has, with her openness, meant a lot to me and I hope that our dialogue will continue.

Ingela,

I am standing in the kitchen making a pie. The children are playing on the lawn, I can hear them laughing. It is three and a half years to the day since Alexander was born. I think of the years which have passed by, at times kneading the dough with a heavy hand. Alexander would have fitted in well with the two out there, I can almost see him taking part in their play. Alexander is everywhere and nowhere. He does not cry out for me as during the first years. The need to visit his grave is no longer as strong. Do you know, I sometimes woke during the night because someone called out, 'Mam!'; it was not Peter and my movement was towards the window.

Possibly Alexander is in Peter's Nangijala. Somewhere I have an invisible bond to something. Naturally he and I will meet, it would be the only meaning with death. Previously I would have thought it silly to think like that, but now it seems so obvious. I now have Alexander; I 'go' to him and come back again. Back from Alexander is everyday-life, where he is not with us.

Now, when I look back, I realise how paralysed we were. A long time. How our thoughts and feelings were filled with what had happened, and how difficult it was to share our experiences with others. Today I wish that those relationships and situations could have been handled differently. But I see it also in the light of others' wish for us soon to be back to normal again.

I believe that nobody understood that time had stopped and refused to start again. We hardly understood, ourselves, how things had to be allowed to run their course. Everything had to go so quickly. As soon as possible we should be back at work again, as if that were a parameter for 'normal life'. Today I wish that we had not bothered with all that but tried to live in our motionless time interval and tried to listen to what it was trying to say to us. It was as though everyone was trying to get away from Alexander. Everyone. Even today I meet people who think that the healing process is the same as forgetting. With this definition I am 'unfledged', as I think about him as much as I do about the other children.

It may seem burdensome to have a dead child in one's heart but it does not weigh me down. Alexander is our snowflake who melted and fell on our shoulders, light as a feather: A little, naked boy sliding down the rainbow.

I am glad that I have had this contact with you, Ingela. You broke my feeling of isolation and of being different. You are the first person I have met who also has given birth to a stillborn child. It was a relief finally to talk to someone like myself.

In my diary I have written, 'Oh Alexander, your beating heart and everything would have been different'. But it was not to be and we have changed. I am still getting to know the person I have become. Often I like her more than the person I was.

The day we buried Alexander, when all that we wished for was to feel his heartbeat, I believed that I could never be happy again. Never properly happy. I am not so certain now. It is true that I cry more easily than before Alexander's death but I also feel that I shall find it easier to laugh.

Warmly,
Maria

To our daughter

Your Mother's joy
spreading news of your existence
even before the laboratory's result
breasts tighten, bleeding stops,
'we are expecting, we are expecting'

You gave us joy by existing
on ultra-sound your contours
for us so beautiful
Your heart beating so regularly
Your arms' movements

You gave us joy by growing
Your Mother's fine stomach
Your strong kicks
did you notice our happy laughter
at your sudden gambols?

And you have heard five languages
heard a large town's clamour, the fells' silence
did you notice the difference in the strides?
The streets' hard asphalt, the forest's embracing snow,
the springy heather of the moors

And I played for you
your Mother sitting securely, knitting
were you listening?
You could hear beautiful ballads, raucous be-bop
and from the gramophone the finest symphonies

Your death, so pointless, so cruel
Your brittle short life
extinguished,
ran out into the surrounding sea
Our beloved child you died

You shall always be a white carnation
sorrowful but beautiful, grief but also joy
Our pride when you were born
our deep despair
tears which emptied each spiritual reservoir

You were so sweet with your fine black hair
Your Mother lifted your chin, 'she has your mouth'
and tenderness welled up within us
I counted your fingers, toes — five
Our tears, grief but also joy

You shall always be a white carnation
the flower we laid to wither on your breast.

Your Father

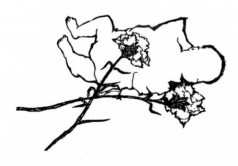

The poem was written by Ellen's father, Gunnar Steineck, the night after her birth.

43

Our Mårten

My name is Karin and I have four children. Mårten, my
third child, would have had his fifth birthday a few weeks
ago if he had lived. Mårten was born and died at the same
time. I felt well while carrying Mårten, but towards the
end I was larger than during previous pregnancies and had
felt more contractions. When there were still five weeks
left to the birth I had sudden, strong pains and had to go
to the hospital. On the labour ward I was given a drip in
an attempt to stop the contractions. The birth continued
even so, and it was decided to let the baby come even if
it was too early. I remember the feeling of sadness when
the paediatrician told me that the baby would be placed
in an incubator after the birth. I was thinking, 'No, I don't
want to be here any longer. I'll go home and come back
when it's time for the birth; the proper birth.'

The incision

The midwife placed a fetal monitor on my stomach to
register the baby's heartbeat. After a while she discovered
that the sounds from the baby indicated distress. A doctor
was called. 'This baby isn't feeling well, we'll have to
help it out', said the doctor. Suddenly the room was full

of people. I was not worried. They were about to help the baby out and I fully trusted the staff. I never understood that my son was so poorly.

Coming to

When I came to after the operation I had the feeling that my husband, Lennart, was close by. He was very quiet. I did not dare think the thought, but felt that something was not quite right. 'He didn't make it', said Lennart. I fell back into a sort of sleep. It could not be true, what Lennart had said. My thoughts went back and forth, things were not as Lennart had said.

To see him

When I woke up, a nurse asked if I wished to see the baby. My reaction was, 'Hell no, how disgusting to see one's dead baby'. I thought of horror stories of dead people suddenly opening their eyes and sitting up. I had, for a while, worked on a labour ward and in a room had seen some strange aluminium boxes. When I asked what they were used for they replied, 'We place the dead babies in the boxes'. I was terrified that they would bring my baby in one of those boxes. When I hesitated about seeing my baby, the nurse told me of parents who had not seen their child and later got it into their heads that someone had stolen it. Then I thought that it would be best to see him any way. A doctor told me that the baby's stomach was swollen; I said to the staff that I only wanted to see his face.

The midwife who had attended the operation came in to us with the baby, he lay in a little bed wrapped in a green sheet. I had mixed feelings when I saw him. All the time I had to convince myself that it was true that he was dead, yet at the same time I was unable to comprehend that it was true. 'He looks as though he is sleeping', said the midwife. All the while I had the feeling that this was not my baby, it should be nothing like this. I had come to the hospital to have a baby, a living baby, and not to look at a dead baby. The midwife asked if I wished to hold the baby but I did not even dare to touch him. I looked at him but could not really see that this was my child. It was my child but at the same time not, since it was a dead child. It was the first and only time that I saw Mårten.

The real awakening

Two days later, when my head started to clear, the feeling that I wanted to see him again grew. It was a conscious decision, and a desire to see *my* child and not a *dead* child which was the feeling that I had the first time that I saw Mårten. I asked the doctor, who came to inform me of the result of the post-mortem, if I could see my child again. The doctor was unable to say yes or no to my request but asked if he could come back after consulting someone else. When the doctor returned the next day he asked how much I remembered of Mårten. I told him that I remembered the eyes, nose, mouth, the little tongue, the hair and forehead. 'In that case, that'll have to do', was the doctor's answer. 'What, has he changed that much,

47

does he look strange now?', I wondered. 'The memory that you have will have to do', was the only answer that I received.

I could not get the thought out of my mind of what they could have done to my child, seeing that they thought that I should be spared from seeing him again. My imagination ran wild and I imagined that they had done the most awful things to him during the post-mortem. Had they possibly cut his face? I imagined the stomach very large and swollen. Then I accepted that they were right to prevent me from seeing him and I did not take up the question again.

The funeral

I think that it was the medical social worker who first spoke to us about the funeral. My first thought was, 'Funeral, are you out of your minds? You can't bury a little child.' However we quite quickly came to think it obvious that Mårten was to be buried and that Lennart and I would be there. I felt that I must take something with me to Mårten's funeral. Red roses, to me a symbol of love, would be right. I thought about how many roses we should take with us. Mårten lived 35 weeks in my stomach. Should I buy 35 roses? It seemed a lot, so I settled on 15 roses since he was born on the fifteenth of the month. The market-gardener was shut on the day of the funeral, even so Lennart managed to get him to open, but he rushed home with fifteen red tulips! In the confusion Lennart had not remembered that I had said roses. I did not know what to do now. Could I ask Lennart to buy some more flowers? Lennart arranged to change the flowers with the obliging gardener, and returned with my red roses. I laid the roses on Mårten's coffin in place of the normal floral tributes, for me it was important that they were our flowers which lay on the coffin. It was our gift to Mårten.

I remember worrying if Mårten was content in his coffin. The coffin seemed so small and cramped. The priest calmed me and said that the woman who laid out children always did so with great care. It was nice to hear. I thought of seeing Mårten again when I saw the coffin, and I asked the priest if it were possible to open the lid. The priest said that it would not be a problem, but then I did not dare to. My fear was based on the fact that I did not quite know what I would see and that I was afraid of getting a poorer memory of Mårten than I had. The doctor's words rang in my ears, 'The memory that you have will have to do'. I cried a lot in the church, quietly weeping, the tears just flowed. It was difficult to imagine that in that small coffin lay our child. It felt comforting to sit there in the small chapel and just let the tears flow.

The cemetery

We decided to have Mårten buried in the children's sacred garden. The reason for not chosing a separate grave with a memorial stone was that we believed that it would become somewhere for which we had a bad conscience, because we did not tend it better. Our expectation of the future was that Mårten would become a distant memory, an episode way back in time for which we would not feel a lot. Today we know that that is not what has happened. One is never 'finished' with what has passed, one never leaves the memories behind. Today we know that we will hold on to the memories we have of Mårten. A separate grave would possibly have helped us to preserve his memory.

Unfortunately we were not allowed to be present at his interment. 'It isn't part of our routine', was the answer, when we asked the verger. I would very much have liked to know in which part of the children's sacred garden Mårten was intered, but they would not tell us that either. I find it very frustrating not knowing exactly where Mårten was buried.

Two weeks after the funeral I took a walk in the cemetery. I looked for the spot where I believed Mårten lay buried. After a while I came to a place covered by a green tarpaulin and a corrugated steel sheet. It was approximately one and a half metres square. Was Mårten lying under under the tarpaulin? I did not dare to lift the tarpaulin to see, I was afraid of finding several coffins stacked, one above the other. I walked a long time in the cemetery going through agonies. What was under the green tarpaulin? I could not get the thought out of my mind that Mårten possibly lay in a mass grave and that other parents had been similarly afflicted. It was enough that we had lost our child; that the same thing had happened to others was more than I could bear. When I came home I told Lennart what I had seen at the cemetery. Lennart went to the children's garden, lifted the steel sheet and the tarpaulin and had a look. All that he saw was earth.

After the funeral I often went to the cemetery. On each visit I had a strong feeling of unreality. I searched for my child, he was there somewhere and yet not, since I did not know where he was buried. I had not had verbal contact with Mårten so it was not like when an older person has died, when one can sit by the gravestone and talk to the deceased. I missed having a fixed spot where I could feel that Mårten was lying here. During the All Souls festival we went to the garden of remembrance and lit a candle and since then I can accept Mårten's sacred garden. If others can have their relatives buried in a garden of remembrance then we can have Mårten in the children's sacred garden.

Facing up to everyday life again

I stayed in hospital for just over a week after the operation. I remember standing by the window in my room on the ward, seeing all the blissful parents leaving the maternity unit with their newly-born babies in small carry-cots. I could also see the motorway outside my window, people travelling in their cars to and from work. I was surprised by how life went on as if nothing had happened.

Coming home again without one's baby is silence. Unreality. Just recently I had had a large stomach, now it was empty and flat. It would be easy to deny that I have ever been pregnant, I could wear my old clothes and there was nothing in the house which could be connected to having a baby. Once home again I felt that I wanted to do something new, my new life should begin. I went jogging a lot, pushing myself more and more on the forest track. At the same time I was angry, words of anger went round in my head while I was running.

We had friends who had babies at the same time as we had Mårten. We lost contact with one couple. They thought that meeting us was awkward. When things were difficult after Mårten's death nobody asked me how I felt, they asked Lennart instead, 'How is Karin?'. When Lennart answered honestly that I was not feeling so well, nobody asked further, there was a silence. Something which I have learnt through Mårten's death is to be brave enough to speak to anyone who is having a difficult time.

Our children have acccepted Mårten's death as natural. Per, who was five when Mårten died, wondered why his young brother had died. We explained as well as we could and told him that Mårten's heart had stopped. Per got out the books that we have which show the body, he lay down on the floor and skimmed through until he found the section showing the heart. At nursery school, Per himself told them of his little brother's death. Two years later when Per started school the teacher asked the children to do a drawing of their families. Per drew himself, his little sister Maria, Lennart and me. In the picture I had an enormous stomach. When I asked Per why he had drawn me with such a large stomach he answered, 'Mårten's there, of course'.

Maria often says that her mother has given birth to four children: Per, Maria, Mårten and Linda. The other day Maria said to a friend, 'Today is Mårten's name-day*'. 'Which Mårten?', said the friend. 'Our Mårten', said Maria. 'What do you mean, 'Our Mårten?'. 'He died', answered Maria. 'Oh him', said the friend. We have developed a tradition in the family, we go to the cemetery every All Souls festival and light a candle for our Mårten.

Understanding

When one finds oneself in a crisis, as I did after Mårten's death, one is very sensitive to the attitude of the people around. I believe that I was met with understanding and respect by many, but the occasions when it was otherwise provide distinct memories. I can remember a nurse who was sent to remove the stitches from the operation. I felt uncomfortable from the moment she entered the room. The nurse hardly talked to me, apart from instructions to make her job easier. Her facial expression and body-

* **Name-day**: In Sweden virtually each day of the calendar has been furnished with one or two Christian names. Mårten's day is the 11th of November and on this day people with this name may enjoy a simple celebration. It may also provide someone with a reason to write a few lines to a friend or relative called Mårten.

language gave rise to an icy atmosphere. She was like a stainless steel sink-top. My stomach was sacred to me; I had borne my baby in it. It felt wrong that this callous person should be touching it. Most of all, I wished to ask her to leave and that someone else should take out the stitches. The feeling of subordination that one can endure as a patient prevented me and I felt deeply hurt.

Only rarely was there any peace in the room during the day. There was always someone who had to do the cleaning or carry out some other task. Tears had to be saved for the nights. All red-eyed from crying, I pressed the call-button to ask for some paper handkerchiefs. The nurse who answered asked if I had a cold. All were not equally lacking in understanding. It was lovely to hear a physiotherapist say, 'It's good to cry, one should cry a lot, I do nearly every day'. Possibly one cannot expect sympathy from everybody, but it does feel like contempt for one's feelings when grief is not met with respect. During the funeral, where only Lennart, I, the priest and the organist were present, I noticed that the organist hurried into the church. She did not look at us, did not take off her coat. We got the impression that the funeral did not mean anything to her: she was just routinely running through her usual tunes.

The social worker

Lennart and I had close contact with the medical social worker who visited us on the ward after Mårten's death.

She told us about all the practical things which we had to get done in the immediate future. We decided to meet again after I had been discharged. The social worker urged us to ring her whenever we felt the need. I thought that it was wonderful to be able to use the hospital's resources even though I was no longer an admitted patient. It was so nice to be able to meet someone who actively listened and who told us that what I was feeling and thinking about had also been experienced by others who had suffered such a loss. The social worker could make less dramatic what had become exaggerated because of my unstable emotional state. She prepared me for situations and feelings so that much later some things seemed familiar – déja vu. It was a relief for me to be able to talk without having to sort out my impressions, and to reveal to someone feelings for which I later would not need to feel responsible.

The midwife

'You are welcome to ring me if there is anything you want to know', said the midwife to me before I left the hospital. She gave me her telephone number. When I had been home a week and did not feel very well I rang her. At first I was uncertain and did not want to be a nuisance, possibly she had not meant what she had said? The midwife came to my home and we talked about what had happened. We already had a good relationship since my time at the hospital and it became even better. It was not so much a midwife-patient relationship, more a mutual female interest. I described wandering round the cemetery, my search for Mårten and all the strange dreams I was having at the time. We continued meeting and discovered that we had a lot of interests in common. We still meet frequently and are the best of friends. We do not often talk about Mårten, but he exists as a mutual experience.

A new baby

I asked at the hospital about when it would be medically possible for me to become pregnant again. They said that there was no particular length of time that we need wait, but that our mourning should be allowed to take its course. When I came home I felt that it was totally impossible to consider having a new baby. A year later I felt ready. I thought that I would get pregnant immediately but it was two and a half years before we were expecting again. On getting the result of the pregnancy test I became frightened. I was convinced that there was something wrong with the baby. Mårten's death was due to a malformed liver, so unusual that at the hospital where he was born they had not seen a similar case since 1939. To eliminate as many things as possible which could go wrong during the pregnancy, I decided to take as many tests as were available. A chorionic villus test was taken early in the pregnancy but was unsuccessful so I had an amniocentesis test during the sixteenth week as well. There was a long wait before I received the result. It showed that there was nothing wrong.

During the first half of the pregnancy I was psychologically unpregnant. I felt panic-stricken before going to the maternity clinic again, to sit there pregnant and to describe what had happened the previous time. My pregnancy with Mårten and the birth became so tangible. I was very fearful of going to the labour ward and realised that I must overcome my fear before it was time to give birth to the new baby. I rang the labour ward, described how I was feeling and asked to be allowed to visit and have a look around. For me it was a turning point, getting my fears into perspective and feeling calmed. I was also able to see a newly-born baby. That meant a lot. After twenty six weeks I could, for the first time, take part in this new pregnancy which was entirely normal. Linda was born healthy and well formed.

Memories

I have worked sufficiently on my grief for Mårten now. I am satisfied. It is not important that I feel sad now and then. There is every reason for feeling sad when one's child has died. I do not wish to lose that part of my grief. I have become more mature, possibly in a broader sense than other people of my age. Previously I was very sensible and emotionally restricted. Through Mårten I have experienced feelings which I did not believe I had.

Mårten's father's thoughts

Staff charge into the delivery room to look after my wife and our baby which is on its way into the world. The midwife has earlier said that the baby is probably not well and therefore needs help to come out quickly. The whole situation is frantic and I feel that I am getting in the way for all these useful people. My wife with the child in her womb is wheeled out of the room to be hurriedly transported to surgery. I remain in the room. Until a moment ago it was an inferno, now it is silent and inhospitable. I stand there with all my thoughts. What is going to happen now? A thought flashes through my mind, what can God do in a situation such as this? I try to eliminate the thought from my mind, feeling anxiety spread through my body. A lump forms in my throat.

I want our third, longed-for, child. We have previously said that if it is a boy he will be called Mårten. We have not discussed a girl's name yet. The door opens and a nurse asks if I would like anything to eat or drink. I thank her, no, but ask if I may stay in the delivery suite. That is no problem. Minutes pass by, they seem like hours. Time seems endless, I have a feeling of helplessness and disappointment within me. Why doesn't anybody tell me how things are going?

The door opens again and the surgeon enters. He informs me that our beloved Mårten did not survive. Unfortunately the doctor can not say any more just now but promises to come back later. I never see him again. In my despair I wonder if the doctor does not dare to return.

The midwife who went with Karin to the operation comes in and tells me what I already know. I spontaneously feel a warmth from someone who cares. I dare to show my disappointment. The midwife wonders if I would like to see Mårten. Initially it seems a strange question but on reflection I wish to see my child who has so hastily left us.

Karin and I have had Mårten amongst us for several months. It has seemed as though the family has consisted of five people. Mårten has been among us like a dream, an illusion, and at the same time existed alongside our other children. It has always been easy to drift into our dreams about Mårten. The similarities to our other children have previously seemed obvious. His room is already ready. Karin has made plans to stay at home with him during her maternity leave. Because of the time of year, Mårten will be able, right from the start, to have his morning and afternoon sleep in the garden. It seems such a privilege, a large family enjoying life together. We have planned the future, expecting Mårten to be coming home.

I answer, 'Yes', when I am asked if I would like to see Mårten; it is obvious that I want to see the boy who has already meant so much to us. The midwife comes in with him wrapped in a towel. He looks to be sleeping. The tears are rolling down my face, I stroke his cheek. When the midwife has taken him out I feel that I would have liked to kiss him on the cheek just like we always kiss our children when it is time for them to go to sleep.

The midwife takes me to Karin and at the same time puts another bed next to her so that we may sleep together. Karin looks at me with sedated eyes. We say nothing to each other. Later, during the night, Karin asks, 'Things didn't go well, did they?'. From my silence she has understood what has happened.

When I come home from the hospital I feel only a great emptiness. My mother, Mårten's grandmother, is sitting in our kitchen and is reading the newspaper. When I have told her what has happened she goes back to reading the paper. At eleven o'clock I fetch Per from nursery school. I take him into my arms and tell him. 'Dad,' he says, 'it doesn't matter, we can get a new one at Christmas instead'. His reaction feels like a release. 'Dad, why does your voice sound so strange?' he asks. I answer that I am very sad.

Telephone conversations with friends and acquaintances are difficult and sad. During some I become so disappointed that I want to throw down the receiver. The first calls cause the most tears but in time calls become more and more mechanical. Friendship is tested at times like this.

Life must continue despite everything. Mårten cannot stay at the hospital. We have to decide if he is to be buried or cremated. These are new questions for us, neither Karin nor I have previously lost a close relative. We feel lost and would prefer it if someone at the hospital could help us with the answers. Unfortunately everybody avoids answering these questions which are so important to us. We feel isolated. Grief and disappointment are sufficiently painful. We do not want other people to make decisions for us, but we want them to tell us what we should not do. What is normal and what is not. The hospital's chaplain finally helps us out of our uncertainty. Only Karin, I and the chaplain are present at the funeral. Karin lays the roses on the coffin lid. The family feels smaller now than it did before Karin was expecting Mårten.

Now, later, I feel that what we have been through has welded us together. I have experienced something which even today, five years later, can make me cry. Previously tears have not fallen naturally for me. I have had a psychological block which has been released.

Life has been given other qualities and does not feel as obvious as before.

Daring to try again

Birgitta and Henrik have, at the time of writing, two months left to the birth of their second baby. Hedvig, their first baby, was born and died fifteen months earlier. Here they describe their time with Hedvig.

Hedvig was born with a large diaphragmatic hernia. The organs in her stomach pushed up into her chest cavity, with the result that her lungs were too small and she could not survive outside the womb. That things were not as they should be was first discovered during the last weeks of pregnancy. Before that everything was normal. At the last visit to the doctor it was decided that Birgitta should have some extra tests, her stomach had suddenly become so large. There was a suspicion that something was wrong. The examinations indicated that everything was normal. With two weeks left to the expected birth, Birgitta was admitted to an antenatal ward. Ultrasound examinations were carried out and concern increased that the baby was deformed. They did not tell us what they suspected to be wrong. During the rounds after an examination Birgitta asked the doctor why her stomach was so large and why there was so much amniotic fluid. 'It can be an indication that there is a malformation', said the doctor.

Birgitta: *I just wanted to get away from there. I asked to be allowed to go home and be discharged. Henrik was at work and I cried all the way home.*

We had a referral letter for yet another ultrasound examination at another hospital where we had an appointment the next day. After a long ultrasound examination the doctor discovered the diaphragmatic hernia. He could not say how large the hernia was.

Birgitta: *I shielded myself. I did not want to think about things not going well. A few days later, when I was on my way to hospital because of the contractions, I was thinking, 'There is nothing wrong with this baby'. We already knew that there was a diaphragmatic hernia. I supressed thoughts of anything wrong. As I walked along the hospital corridor feeling the contractions and looking forward to giving birth, I thought that everything would be all right as long as the baby came out.*

The contractions declined but we were allowed to sleep at the hospital overnight. The next day it had been decided that we should go to a children's hospital where Birgitta was to have a Caesarean section. The baby could then be quickly operated on if it were necessary. Meta came and introduced herself as our midwife, she was to follow us to the hospital.

Henrik: *Everything then went very quickly. Birgitta was anaesthetised and I had to stay outside the operating theatre. I saw them rush out from there carrying a small bundle. After a while a doctor came and told me that the baby girl was not so well. At first I did not want to go in and look at her in the incubator, I was afraid. Meta and the paediatrician almost had to force me to go in to take a look at my daughter. I was terrified when I looked down at her. She was obviously very poorly.*

Birgitta: *When I awoke after the operation Henrik came in to me and told me that we had a baby girl and that she was very poorly. I cannot recollect how I reacted at the time. I still had a lot of anaesthetic in me and I felt drowsy.*

Henrik: *The paediatrician asked if we were going to baptise our baby. We had not had a thought of having her baptised but, after thinking it over for a while, it felt the right thing to do.*

Three hours after the operation Hedvig was baptised. It was the first time that Birgitta saw her daughter.

Birgitta: *I was not fully awake. I remember looking at the priest who was to baptise Hedvig, he looked afraid. Hedvig was so small, she lay in the incubator with tubes and wires stuck to her body. Everything was unreal. It felt like a dream. I felt that I should cry but I could not. My body did not obey the feelings which were inside me.*

The intention was that Birgitta was to return to the first hospital when she had come round after the operation. We were at a children's hospital and they did not want to take responsibility for Birgitta so soon after the operation. Because the ambulance which was to take us back was delayed, we had the opportunity to see Hedvig again. Meta did not give Birgitta any pain-relief and that made her more awake and more aware of things.

Hedvig died at twenty minutes to one that same night.

Birgitta: *I regret now that I was not able to stay at the hospital and be there when she died. I would very much have liked to hold Hedvig in my arms while she was still warm. The staff must have known that she was going to die. They could have taken her out of the incubator, removed the tubes and cables and let Hedvig die with me. I was almost certain that she was going to die that night, but at the same time I tried to suppress the thought. I remember saying to Meta when we were travelling back in the ambulance, 'When do you think that we can try again? I want to have a lot of children, I want to have a lot of children!'*

Henrik: *In contrast to Birgitta I was fully conscious during and after Hedvig's birth. I had understood part of the staff's conversation with each other concerning Hedvigs's chances of survival. From what I had heard, Hedvig was in a serious condition. I pressured the paediatrician, wanted my suspicions confirmed. The paediatrician told me and I could draw the conclusion myself that Hedvig would not survive but that it was impossible to say how long she would live. It felt comforting to get confirmation. Now, later, I think that it was unfortunate that Hedvig's condition did not improve for a few days as it sometimes can. We would then have had time to get used to the idea of what was going to happen.*

Late that night Henrik went home, he was restless and could not sleep.

Henrik: I *looked in the books we read while we were expecting Hedvig. Books about giving birth and what it is like to have a baby. In one of the books there was a chapter on having a miscarriage and babies which die. We had skipped over those pages when we had previously read the book. That will not happen to us, we thought then. I now read the chapter and when, during the night, they rang from the hospital and said that Hedvig had died, it was something that I was prepared for.*

Birgitta: *When I awoke in the morning I had a dreadful, strong feeling, 'Hedvig is not alive'. At the same time I was not entirely certain. I rang home to Henrik and he confirmed it.*

Birgitta and Henrik shared a room on the ward.

Birgitta: *The staff were wonderful. Nobody avoided us, rather we felt that they cared about us. One day, when I was feeling very sad and was brooding over why this should happen to us, a nurse sat down on the edge of the bed. The nurse held me in her arms and even she was crying. Her sympathy warmed me.*

The next day, the paediatrician who was on duty when Hedvig died, rang. He asked if we wished to come to the hospital and see her again. We had not thought that we would be able to do that, and at the same time were afraid to go there. We asked Meta if she would be able to come with us.

We met the paediatrician in his room and he told us why Hedvig died, that it was an unusual malformation and that it was just chance that she was stricken. We went together to a chapel and the paediatrician brought Hedvig. She was lying in a small bed. It was all unreal but our nervousness and anxiety disappeared as soon as Hedvig came into the room. We sat a long time with our daughter.

When the paediatrician was to return her to the mortuary he stopped by the door and said, 'You may hold her, Birgitta'. Just at that moment I was feeling that it was what I wanted to do, but I did not dare. Both Henrik and I held her in our arms and I felt so calm afterwards.

On returning to our room on the ward we now felt able to ring our friends and relatives to tell them what had happened.

The funeral

The funeral was held in the chapel at the hospital. Our parents were there. We had arranged flowers and wreaths with which we adorned the coffin. It looked so nice. The priest was the same one who had baptised Hedvig. He said such beautiful words to Hedvig and to us. The funeral is a lovely memory. Later we placed Hedvig's urn in the garden of rest, this time there were only we two present. We read a poem for our child.

Let us be silent
a moment together
let us listen
in wordless harmony
let us open slightly the door
to a secret room
where the soul is
still and free
where the world's pulse
can not reach
where neither worry nor time can reach
be still
and listen together
to tones
which the world does not know
be still
and strength shall flow
from the spring
of
eternity

The Shepherd Girl, from Poems by Barbro Karlén. Zindermans 1972.

The time after Hedvig's funeral

We talked a lot and became very close in the time which followed. The medical social worker and our paediatrician gave us wonderful support. We planned a trip abroad and thought of getting married at the same time.

Birgitta: *It helped me during the time when I was off work sick to have something to take my mind off things. I planned the trip abroad and the arrangements concerning the wedding.*

Henrik: *What was most disturbing afterwards was that Birgitta changed jobs when she started work again. That meant that she came into contact with a lot of people who did not know what had happened to us. It was unfortunate to expose oneself to that just then.*

Birgitta: *At times I felt so strong but then, from out of the blue, the ache in the chest; an enormous sorrow which swept over me.*

The decision about a new pregnancy

Henrik: *Birgitta had already asked while in the hospital when it would be suitable to plan a new pregnancy. We were given the advice to wait until mid-summer, Hedvig was born in February. We began I supppose before then but Birgitta did not start to menstruate.*

Birgitta: *Things were difficult. I could not run to the antenatal clinic every time that I thought that I was pregnant. I went to my doctor and asked to be given hormones to start off my menstrual cycle again but she refused.*

In August Birgitta started to menstruate again, but did not become pregnant.

Birgitta: *In November I had an appointment for an examintion. I felt that they now really did have to help me in some way. I sat in the doctor's surgery feeling sorry for myself because I had not become pregnant. Then she asked, 'When did you last have a period?'. I explained that it was certainly one and a half months back. I gave a urine sample and a pregnancy test was carried out. The test showed that I was pregnant. I did not understand a thing. It took a few days before I could accept that I was pregnant. The immediate joy quickly turned to anxiety. It was nice to be told that I was pregnant; now I knew that my body was working again. At the same time I was very fearful of having a miscarriage; 'This'll never work out', I thought.*

At the end of November Birgitta started suddenly to bleed. She was having a meal in a restaurant with a friend. Henrik was away on a trip, abroad. Birgitta went straight to Meta. After an examination Birgitta's anxiety was calmed, it was not a miscarrriage. The bleeding was small and had already stopped.

Birgitta: *The whole pregnancy has been unsettled, obviously I have been happy now and then but anxiety was always close to the surface. Can it really work out this time? After the first three* months, when there is the greatest risk of a miscarriage, came the fear that the baby would be born prematurely. I have never thought that the baby would suffer from the same thing as Hedvig, but that there would be something else wrong.

Henrik: *Birgitta asked to have the same midwife and paediatrician during the new pregnancy as we had for Hedvig, and that has been agreed to. Some extra examinations have even been carried out.We have also contacted our social worker again when we got the message that we were expecting once more.We feel that everyone is really giving us their support.*

People's reaction to the new pregnancy

Birgitta: *For the most part friends and acquaintances believe, seeing it is such a long time since Hedvig died and that we are expecting again, that we have got over what happened. They seem to believe that we have forgotten Hedvig and that we have finished grieving.*

Henrik: *People often say to me, 'Now Birgitta must be feeling well – when you are expecting a baby again'.*

Birgitta: *Then they are shocked when I am sad and can still cry over what happened. There is a conflict within me. I am very pleased about the new baby but still mourn Hedvig.*

Thinking about Hedvig

Birgitta: *I think about Hedvig every day. I think about how things went at the hospital, how things would have been if she* had survived. A fantasy. I can sometimes feel so despairing because I did not get the chance to get to know her.

Henrik: *When I see parents with children who have just learnt to walk, I usually think that Hedvig would also be doing that now.*

During the nights since Hedvig's death Birgitta has had many dreams and her anxiety during the new pregnancy has resulted in even more dreams.

Birgitta: *Most of the dreams are about my having a baby. The birth is always skipped over, I just have a baby. In one dream I go into town. I walk for a long time, looking around. I want to buy a dummy but all the shops are shut. My stomach is very large.*

At the end of the day I take the underground home. I ring Henrik from the station. He tells me then that we have a child. We have a little girl and when I hear that my large stomach disappears. I am suddenly thin again.

Another dream is about when I am picking flowers in a large meadow. When I come home with my bouquet we have had a baby. There are two girls, one is a baby and the other is about three years old. They were just there in the house when I got home.

I have also had many dreams about having babies which are dead or live a while and then die. Many dreams include deformed babies, they have boils and deformed arms.

Once I dreamed that I was looking after my brother's baby, which is three months old. When I come out into the garden to take a look at him when he is sleeping, I find him dead.

Possibly the most vivid dream that I have had is when I am about to get a dog. I am exhilarated and happy because I shall be able to choose one for myself. The dogs are in a row of small white cardboard boxes, they look like small white coffins. I decide which box I want. When I lift the lid to take a look at my dog I see that he is lying in the bottom of the box. The dog is dead. This dream troubled me for several days.

Another very unpleasant dream I have had is about a visit to a friend. In the dream she is getting ready to move. My friend wants to have one of the rooms decorated completely in marble. Marble is expensive so instead of buying some she has taken marble gravestones from the cemetery. She has put up gravestones everywhere in the room, the walls and floor are covered. I wander round her new flat. In one room I discover the priest who buried Hedvig. He is very angry and regrets that he cannot spend as much time as he would like with his own children. He tells us that he has no time to spare for us.

I also remember a dream I had shortly after Hedvig died. I was flying on my own. I was flying at low level and it was going really well despite the fact that I did not have any wings. I described the dream for our social worker and she interpreted it as a symbol that I would get over my grief. She thought that I should take Henrik with me the next time that I went flying.

Feelings before the birth of the new baby

Henrik: *I push the thought of it to one side now, unlike last time. Then I wanted to find out as much as possible. How the birth is going to take place is less important now, the main thing is that we keep the baby. At the same time I am worried and think of how things will be if all does not go well. There are those who take several blows like this in life. We cannot be certain that we will be spared this time either. I wonder if we can survive another experience like this?*

Birgitta: *Sometimes I am certain that things will go well, and then I become frightened because I have such positive thoughts. Ever since I became pregnant I have wished that the birth would take place today. I want to know now how it will end. To avoid the months of waiting in uncertainy. Last time everything was so new. I cannot say that I think that it is especially pleasant to be pregnant now. Friends give cheery greetings, 'How big you are now Birgitta!'. To me the word 'big' is negatively charged. I know that I must not become too large. That was what happened last time when there was too much amniotic fluid. That was how they discovered that there was something wrong. I do not like it when they say that my stomach is large. I know that most of those who say that have no idea what happened last time, even so I do not like to hear it said. Some who know what it was like last time can still say, 'It looks as though you are going to be just as big as last time, Birgitta'. They cannot imagine what it is like to be in my situation.*

What will it be like when the new baby is born?

Henrik: *I envisage that we will over-protect the baby. What has gone before is going to characterize our relationship with our child. Possibly it will be a disadvantage but one cannot tell.*

Birgitta: *We are not planning anything now. That is what we did the last time. We are not buying any baby clothes or a pram. We still have the clothes intended for Hedvig, but we returned the pram to the shop. This time there will be no pram bought before there is a baby to lay in it. Even so I do not regret buying things for Hedvig, I got pleasure out of it then.*

Henrik: *I often think about whether it will be a boy or a girl. I hope that it will be a girl. I do not know if I really mind or whether I have been influenced by Birgitta's very strong desire to have another girl. In one way, if it is a boy it will not be so easy to identify him with Hedvig. If it is a girl then I think that it will be easier to compare her with Hedvig. I am not sure that it would be such a good thing.*

Birgitta: *The main thing is that the baby is healthy, then it does not matter what it is. Obviously I think that it will be a girl. Hedvig was of course a girl.*

What Hedvig has meant

Henrik: *I do not take anything for granted any more. I have become calmer. What I used to react strongly to, and to think important, does not mean as much today.*

Birgitta: *I understand people who are afflicted by grief. I have been given a treasure, one which I would have preferred to be without and instead been able to keep Hedvig.*

A change in our relationship since Hedvig's death

Henrik: *I think that our relationship has acquired a deeper level of contact. I see our relationship as more obvious today, and I have difficulty in imagining that I could live any other way.*

Birgitta: *We have a strong background, Henrik and I. We have discussed so much together during this time and have become very close.*

After the second baby's birth

Birgitta and Henrik had a son two months after our conversation. Three months later the following was written.

Henrik: *Our anxiety before the birth became greater the nearer the expected day came. When it finally started we felt a great security. Meta was with us the whole time. As midwife and friend, Meta has meant a great deal to us, she has helped us through this difficult time. Meta got us to believe that all would turn out well this time. She helped make the delivery a fine occasion which, when things were at their darkest, we never thought we would be able to enjoy.*

Birgitta: *I get such a wonderful tingling feeling which spreads a warmth throughout my body when I think of our baby boy who is three months old now. I recognise it from the time after Hedvig's birth and death but then the feeling was transformed into anguish and pain instead of warmth. I could never encounter the feeling and pick up and hold Hedvig. Now I can satisfy the need which is expressed by that feeling. I bend over, look at my baby, pick him up and hold him in my arms.*

Be close, listen and be there...

Meta has worked as a midwife for eighteen years. She works on the maternity ward of a large hospital where there are about four thousand births a year. Meta has helped bring several thousand babies into the world in her years as a midwife. We met one day to talk about what one, as a midwife, can go through when a baby dies.

What were you taught during your training about how one helps at a delivery where the baby is stillborn?
I cannot recollect that it was ever mentioned. At least, there was nothing that made a lasting impression on me. During my training I was never present at a delivery where the baby was stillborn. I saw dead babies but I was never the midwife.

Can you remember what it was like the first time that you assisted at the delivery of a stillborn baby?
I cannot remember the first one but I can remember how we worked when I was newly qualified as a midwife. We tried to ensure that the mother saw and experienced as

79

little as possible of the delivery. The father was not usually present. Our primary aim was always to ensure that the mother should not suffer pain unnecessarily. Pethidine and valium were combined. Gas and air was used a lot. In contrast to today's local anaesthetics, the anaesthetics in use then affected the mother's level of consciousness and often she was heavily sedated during the delivery. At the end, when the baby was just about to emerge, the mother was fully anaesthetised. She was given what was called 'final anaesthetic', or a large amount of gas. Even women giving birth to live babies were given anaesthetic, but when it was known that the baby was stillborn it was considered even more important that this was effective. The baby was quickly hidden under green sheets after delivery and then hurriedly taken into the sluice room. When it had been weighed and measured, the baby was taken away in an aluminium box by a porter. By the time the mother recovered from the anaesthetic it was almost all tidied away.

We thought that we were doing it right!

Because the mother was so heavily anaesthetised during the delivery we did not talk to her very much. The attitude then was not to talk about it afterwards either. It was thought best for the mother to know as little as possible. We should not stir things up, so that she would more easily get over what had happened and the best thing was to have another baby as soon as possible.

It was the doctor's job to inform the parents if there was anything wrong with the baby, we midwives were not allowed to do that. This meant that if a deformed baby was born, it was quickly removed from the room while the midwife stayed in the room with the mother, but she could not say anything about what was wrong. There was an awful wait many times. I very soon broke the rule about not saying how the baby was and what could be wrong. If the baby died after the birth or was stillborn it was the doctor's job to show the parents the dead baby, we midwives were not allowed to take any initiative. Most often the parents were not allowed to see their baby. We thought we were doing right when we swept it all under the carpet.

After the delivery the mother was taken to a gynaecological ward. The parents were informed that the hospital would take care of the burial. From my colleagues I learned that the stillborn babies were normally buried together with a deceased adult. The dead baby was laid on the arm of the adult and by that means the baby was buried in consecrated ground. The parents were not, as a rule, told where the baby was buried.

Meta, how do you work today and what do you think is important for the care of parents who lose their baby?
The care that we give today can hardly be compared to what was given even just fifteen years ago. What I know

about how we best should support parents in this situation has mostly been learnt from the mothers and fathers I have met through the years. One of the occasions when I recognised the importance of parents seeing their baby was through a couple with whom I came into contact five years ago. It was a mother who during delivery had to undergo an emergency Caesarean section. The baby died during the operation. The next day a nurse rang from the ward where the mother was an in-patient, they wanted the baby brought up so that the mother could see him.

To show the parents, the next day, a baby which has died is not something for which, at that time, I would have taken the initiative. On the other hand, to me it seemed natural for the parents to see their child about the time of the delivery. I was pleased that the mother wished to see her child and I placed the boy in a bed and took him to the parents. When I got there I held the baby in my arms and showed him to them. The mother stayed on the ward a while because of the operation and it seemed natural to visit her from time to time. The parents expressed several times how much they appreciated that I had picked up their son and held him in my arms, just as with a live baby. The way that I held the boy was not something I had thought about or was conscious of myself. I understand now how much parents see and notice things which can be important to them much later. For this mother and father it felt nice and comforting that their baby was treated caringly.

She kissed her daughter on the forehead

Another two parents from whom I have learnt a lot are Birgitta and Henrik who describe in this book what they went through. I went with them to the children's hospital where the Caesarean section was to be carried out. When the baby came out she looked perfectly healthy, with a nice colour and muscle tone, but she didn't cry. The paediatrician took her to the resuscitation table where she suddenly became worse. She was quickly taken to the special-care baby unit where she was placed in an incubator and ventilator. I stood there in the operating theatre in a strange hospital, without a baby. I did not know what was happening and had no idea whether or not she was going to survive.

Breaking the news

I returned to Henrik who is sitting in a waiting room. A doctor came up to us. He must have been very inexperienced. He did not know how he should tell us the bad news. He had such a hard job keeping his facial expression normal that it looked as though he was smiling. Henrik and I reacted in the same way, we leapt up from the sofa where we were sitting, keen to hear good tidings. She was going to make it! I shall never forget the feeling when the doctor told us that the situation was very serious. 'The baby is very ill', he said, but he still looked as though he was telling us good news.

More like a friend

Henrik was afraid and did not want to go with us to see his baby in the incubator. I took his hand and we went in together to see her. From that moment I was no longer the midwife but more like a friend. The surroundings were strange even for me. I was there in the background, supporting. I made sure that Henrik could ring the grandparents, that he saw Birgitta and that he got something to eat. I knew from previous occasions that a photograph means a lot to the parents so I asked one of the doctors on the ward if they possibly had a camera. It so happened that he had his own camera in his room. He fetched it and bought a film which he gave to the parents. It turned out that he was the doctor who later was to be responsible for their care. I have learnt a lot from him.

The priest knelt amongst cables and tubes

Birgitta and Henrik had their baby baptised a few hours after she was born. The baptism was a beautiful occasion. The priest came in and like all the others present he was wearing a blue gown, it hid his vestments. With him he had a baptismal chalice and candles. Everything stopped in the room. The activity round the other incubators ceased. The priest knelt down and said a prayer by Hedvig's incubator. It was a beautiful service despite the sterile surroundings with machines, hoses, cables and powerful lighting. It was a sight that I never shall forget, the priest kneeling by the incubator.

Back to Hedvig

Late at night, after the baptism, I travelled back to our hospital in the ambulance with Birgitta. Two days later she telephoned me and asked if I would like to go with them back to the children's hospital to see Hedvig, who had died the night after the Caesarean section. I promised to go with them, at the same time feeling some trepidation. Not at the thought of seeing a dead baby, but thinking about the reactions from Birgitta and Henrik.

First we met the doctor who had been on duty on the night when Hedvig had died. He was informative, proper and at the same time humble with regard to what he was telling us. I felt that even I was well taken care of. We were then to go together to the mortuary to see Hedvig. Mostly for the sake of Birgitta and Henrik, I felt uncomfortable about this. On previous occasions when I have been close to a dead baby it has been in connection with the delivery. The baby is still warm and feels almost to be alive. Going down to the mortuary, where the refrigeration fans are continually audible, to see a baby which has lain dead for almost two days was different.

Are you afraid...?

There was a lovely, small chapel next to the mortuary. We waited there while the doctor fetched Hedvig. In the meantime he had prepared Birgitta and Henrik about how a baby which has been dead for some time looks. It is cold, stiff and has a different colour from a live baby. I was intensly aware of Birgitta's apprehension. I asked her, 'Are you afraid, Birgitta?'. 'Yes Meta, I am scared of seeing a dead person', she answered.

The doctor came in with Hedvig in a small bed. That same moment the tense atmosphere in the room changed. It was sad, incredibly sad, but at the same time a wonderful experience. I had a hard job holding back the tears. I cried, but silently, when I saw how naturally and tenderly Birgitta and Henrik accepted Hedvig. They talked to her, saying everything that they had not been able to say to her earlier. Through seeing them then, what they did on seeing their daughter, I felt that this was the right thing to do, so good and important.

Birgitta and Henrik had with them roses from Birgitta's parents, and they told Hedvig who the flowers were from. They also said how sad people were that she had not been allowed to live. Strangely it felt natural to be there. I felt that both the doctor and I were there supporting; it was a private occasion for the parents despite the fact that we were there too. Birgitta and Henrik took photographs of Hedvig. She was so lovely, looking like a doll which was sleeping. There was nothing which was unpleasant or frightening. Birgitta and Henrik relaxed more and more. They asked the doctor about different things, looked at and caressed Hedvig. After a while they were satisfied.

You may hold her...

The doctor was on his way out with Hedvig, but he turned when he reached the door and said, 'You may certainly hold her if you wish, Birgitta'. I know that I felt, 'No don't push her, she cannot manage much more. That's enough. Why does he want to urge her to do that? Hedvig is stiff and cold.' 'Yes, I would like to', said Birgitta cautiously. 'She is a bit stiff and cold', said the doctor before handing over Hedvig to Birgitta. I do not think that she even noticed. Henrik also held her and they took photographs of each other. Birgitta kissed Hedvig on the brow, it was so very beautiful. After a while Birgitta said, 'It feels all right now, I feel well'. Birgitta handed Hedvig over to the doctor.

When we were on our way back to the car the atmosphere was almost of exhilaration. We had done something which was good, and peace reached our hearts. The mood became almost jocular. We had been so tense before the meeting and it felt such a relief that we had coped. I am very pleased that I was be there with them on this occasion. If one has seen the good there is in the contact between parents and their baby then one becomes convinced of how important it is.

Hoping to meet again under different circumstances

I have been in touch with Birgitta and Henrik during the year or so since Hedvig's death. They are not the first parents I have heard express the desire to meet their midwife in more pleasant circumstances. Probably if one has shared such deep sorrow then there is also the desire to share joy.

In a few days Birgitta and Henrik will give birth to their second child. They have asked if I would like to be their midwife and I would very much like to. It feels both exciting and joyful to be able to be there. I know that it means a lot to Birgitta that I shall be there. She is aware that I know what has happened before and therefore she will not need to tell some stranger all about it.

As a professional person it is difficult not to feel that a new baby can be compensation for the baby who died. In a way it is compensation for the unattained role as parents, at least if it is their first baby who has died. I know that they will never want, or be able, to replace Hedvig with a new baby.

I can feel anxiety that something will happen this time. It would be terrible if something were to happen again. But even if something does go wrong I feel that I can help support them. I know that with the birth approaching Birgitta is fearful that there could be another emergency Caesarean section. I understand the reason for her anxiety, and I will try to make things as comfortable as possible even in such a situation.

Does it happen that parents say that they definitely do not wish to see their baby which has died?

It is quite often the first reaction, especially if the baby has been diagnosed as stillborn in the womb. They do not wish to take part any more, they just want to get away. 'Put me to sleep, operate and remove the baby and let me leave here as quickly as possible', is the immediate reaction. The parents often feel panic-stricken before the event but usually calm down if they are given the chance. I can tell you about a couple whose attitude was to see and experience as little as possible, we can call them Eva and Magnus.

Respecting personal integrity

Eva and Magnus came to the labour ward one morning because the womb had been so calm the previous day and during the night. Eva had not felt any movement. We determined that the baby had died, no sound from the baby could be heard and no heartbeat could be seen on an ultrasound scan. The parents' reaction was, 'Quick, help start the delivery so that we can get rid of this thing and go home'. They did not want to leave the ward before the baby had been delivered. It was not Eva's first baby, it was fully developed and everything seemed ready for the delivery, so the doctor decided to start the contractions with an infusion. Eva soon said that she did not wish to see the baby when it was born. I listened and did not argue. At the same time I tried to behave so that nothing was determined in advance. Obviously I had to respect the parents' wishes, but I also had to act in accordance with my own knowledge of what is best in the long term.

I had to take one small step at a time, explaining things. The parents were able to express their conviction about how they wanted things. I let the matter rest, accepting what they said and letting it be that way. In a way I felt that, as time passed, they realised themselves what they really wanted. I possibly led them to a decision which they did not expect to make at the beginning. It seemed natural that things worked out as they did. Because Eva did not wish to see anything, she was moved over to a normal bed after the anaesthetic had been administered, with her in the lithotomy position on the delivery bed. Normally when I deliver a baby with the mother in the lithotomy position I place the baby directly on the mother's stomach. I could not do that this time. There was a reason behind my delivering the baby on the normal bed. Normally, when the baby has come out it lies there a while before the umbilical cord is cut. It is the most natural thing in the world to open one's eyes and take a look, and that is what Eva and Magnus did.

One never regrets later that one has seen one's child

From not wanting to see anything it soon became a matter of course for both of them to see the baby. Things became very still. Time stopped and, despite the anguish, I believe that both felt it to be a fine moment. I believe that it was only when the baby had been delivered that they, for the first time, could understand what had happened. Death only becomes real when the senses can perceive it.

I placed the baby in a bed and not on the mother's arm as I normally do. I felt that it would not be right for these parents. I think that it goes without saying that to see the baby should be a possibility for all, but not a necessity for all. It is necessary to accept that we are all different.

A chance to be alone

After a while, I left the parents alone. They could reach me if they wished to. The baby was there in the room with them. I believe that one must be able to be one's own master a while. However close the relationship between staff and patient, one must still be able to feel, 'Now there are only we two'. After a while I went back in to them. We sat together in the room for quite a while. All their questions came out. I described how the funeral and burial could take place and told them about others I have met who have been in the same situation as themselves. I tried to convey to them that there was no hurry to decide what needed to be done and that they should take their time in considering the alternatives.

Eva and Magnus had a great need to talk and ask questions. I realised that they would not be staying very long at the hospital and therefore I felt that it was especially important for me to answer as many questions as possible. The conversation was a long one. When I came out of the room I met one of my colleagues who asked what on earth I had been doing for such a long time with the parents. My colleague thought that we should take the baby so that it could be prepared and handed over to the porter. It takes time to change working methods. Many old attitudes remain. That I can understand but just then, after such an emotional commitment, it was difficult to accept a reaction like that.

To help just enough

In this sort of situation I think that it is difficult to draw a distinction between professional and private aspects of the job. I cannot do it. Luckily it is so uncommon for a baby to die that it is not usually a problem. It is important that we the staff support one another and help out. When a baby dies it is difficult even for me as a midwife; sometimes powerful emotions are aroused. It is also important that we can decline. At the moment I do not have the strength to participate at the delivery of a stillborn child, I have so many other problems just now and feel that I am unable to give adequate support. If one is new to the job and feels uncertain then one must approach a more experienced colleague for help.

I think that some people feel that a dead baby is not really a baby, a person. Of course it can be difficult with a seriously deformed baby. But it is a baby, the parents' baby. If this happens, it is even more important that the staff behave as naturally as possible towards the baby. On the occasions when babies are deformed, maceration of the skin has occured or they are covered in meconium, it is difficult for parents to approach their own baby. We have to explain to them why the baby looks like it does and show them that it is not dangerous to touch it. My body-language exposes my relationship to the dead baby, I do not believe that we can conceal it. If we feel afraid of contact with a dead baby then we should not take responsibility for those parents who find themselves in this situation.

Can we ever be perfect?

We can never know everything or be a type of professional carer looking after parents bereaved by perinatal death. The backgrounds and needs of the parents vary. I think the most important thing is to listen sensitively. We can acquire knowledge by talking to others and discussing it at work.

Obviously we can devise some guidelines for what one should not forget at the delivery. For example, the parents should see their child, we can gather objects connected with the baby and take some photographs. How this will be done is impossible to say in advance. It is important that we follow up the parents' progress, and that they feel that they can return to us if they wish to. The consequences of each case can not be known until afterwards. If one has had such cases before then obviously it is easier to know how best to help the parents. Most often it is a question of one's own fear, and this shows itself as uncertainty to those parents who possibly have an attitude of rejection. It can be difficult to speak one's mind and advise parents to do things which they possibly will not appreciate until much later. We should indicate the possibilities, but it is the parents who must be in control. We should not intrude or make assumptions. We must not push parents into a fixed schedule and become insensitive to the natural course of events.

It is the parents' right to grieve

There are such strong emotions when a child dies that it is easy to allow oneself to be drawn into this enormous tragedy. As a member of staff, it is still necessary to keep some detachment from what has occurred. It should not happen as in one case I heard of. A small baby died on the maternity ward the night after she was born. The nurse found the baby dead in its bed in the nursery. When she went to inform the mother of what had happened, she was presumably so shocked herself that she was crying hysterically. She had lost all self-control. The mother who had lost her baby had no chance of getting any professional help.

Of course, we may show the feelings we have, and our sympathy, but it is not our pain which is the most important. We have no right to take from the parents their grief.

Meta, how would you like to improve the care which is provided today for those parents who lose their newly-born children?

We have started to talk more about these questions at the hospital where I work. This has led to some very positive changes. In order to improve the cooperation between different categories of staff, we have decided that a midwife, a medical social worker and a doctor should work together as a team to plan the care for each pair of parents. This has resulted in an improvement for us, the midwives. It enables us to maintain contact with parents after the delivery. Previously we have passed on the responsibility to social workers and doctors. I believe that parents need to be able to meet the midwife who was there at the delivery and go through the sequence of events again and again. The increased contact within the staff means that we have a better understanding of one another. It is important that the parents feel that the staff are working together for their sakes.

A contact group provided by the hospital

I would very much to like to help form a contact group for parents who have lost their very young babies. As a midwife I have often been asked, 'Do you know anyone else who has suffered in the same way as we have?'. The contact group could be an opportunity for parents in similar situations to 'find' each other and establish contact. The group's members could change, some turning up only once while others possibly participate for a longer period. Both those who have recently suffered a loss and those for whom it has been a longer time could benefit from meeting. The form of the group could vary depending on the needs of the parents who are taking part at the time. Different people could be associated with the group: a midwife, a social worker, a gynaecologist, a paediatrician, a psychologist, a hospital chaplain. I believe that we, the staff, could learn a lot from such a group. As a midwife, I wish that we would talk more about grief and reactions to crises. We could have day-long meetings to cover a theme where we exchange experiences, listen to lectures and discuss our ideas.

I love my work as a midwife and have never regretted my choice of career even if it has not always been a joy. Even the distressing part of my work has enriched my life and developed me as a person. I feel a greater humility in life. I feel grateful if I, despite the trauma, can help to transform a birth where the baby dies into a fine memory.

Helping to create a precious memory

It is a boundless tragedy when a baby is stillborn or dies shortly after birth. At the same time, it is the birth of a child to which the parents have given life. A child which has developed, grown in the womb and lived in the parents' imaginations for a long time. Now they will meet their long-expected baby, but this meeting requires that they must also say farewell. The staff should contribute in such a way that the meeting, despite the pain, can be a memory for the parents; a memory which also contains something precious. When we are successful, we help the parents to avoid long-term psychological complications of the stillbirth.

In this chapter I attempt to summarise the most important pieces of information from the accounts in the book and, together with knowledge from research, provide guidance about how support for parents should be provided.

Meeting and farewell

'We have two hours, two hours which should have been a lifetime.'

(Letter from Maria)

It is important that the staff should not hasten or interupt the parents' time with the baby. The parents must be allowed to shape the memory they wish to retain. The farewell must not be left incomplete. The parents must themselves decide how long they wish to have together with their dead child, even if it takes several hours or days.

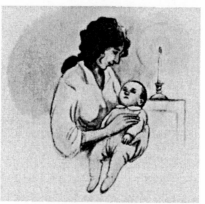

'This one occasion can never be repeated, can never be redone.'

(Letter from Maria)

The staff should neither verbally nor with body-language say anything to the parents so that they dare not look at or touch their child. A well thought-out routine is essential at the delivery of a stillborn child. Do not ask if the parents wish to see the baby, one never asks with a healthy baby. The question implies that it is not a matter of course to see one's dead baby and that can make the parents uncertain. Give the baby to the parents or hold it in your arms in the same way as you would hold a live baby. Large deformities can be concealed. Cover them with clothes or a blanket until the parents are prepared to see them.

A few mothers may refuse to see their child. It is crucial to discuss this reaction immediately – the moment does not come back.

'We place warm blankets around him. We touch him, caress him, he is unbelievably beautiful. We give him a name.' (Letter from Maria)

Tokens of remembrance

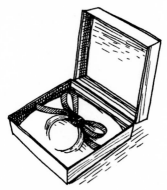

'Just think, if I had a lock of hair from my child; such a priceless treasure!' (said by a woman participating in a long-term follow-up survey)

There is no doubt that a collection of tokens of remembrance from the child is essential for the long-term benefit of the parents. The benefit is documented both statistically and from many women's statements. Directly after birth a photograph should be taken, a lock of hair cut and prints made from a hand and a foot. Try to take the photograph of the baby before the body undergoes post-mortal changes and take care over the arrangement of the picture. A picture of a stillborn child should not be a polaroid snapshot of a dead, unwashed, naked baby on bloody sheets but ideally be a serene picture of a seemingly sleeping child wearing comfortable clothes. Take a picture of the parents together with their baby so that they look like a family. A piece of hair, prints from hands and feet, an ultrasound picture, identity band and birth certificate can also stimulate meaningful memories. The blanket in which the baby was wrapped and the baby's clothes can be saved. Objects related to the baby can be placed in a small box or book of remembrance which is then presented to the parents.

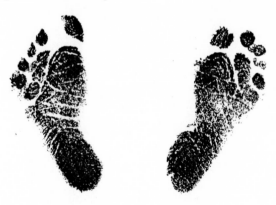

'From not wanting to see anything it soon became a matter of course for both of them to see the baby. Things became very still.'
(Meta in 'Be close, listen and be there...')

Finding the right words

It is impossible to give any advice as to what to say to the parents. On the other hand there are lots of cliches which probably never have the desired effect and which sometimes make the pain worse.

Examples of phrases which should be avoided are:

- The baby would have been abnormal anyway.

- It was for the best the way things worked out.

- The baby was so undeveloped.

- You would never have got to know the baby anyway.

- At least you have other children at home.

- You can always have another baby.

Time for labour induction

There is no scientific support for the practice of delaying labour induction when the baby is dead. Some argue that it is beneficial for the parents to 'digest the trauma' before delivery. My own survey showed that a wait of more than 24 hours was a strong predictor for later anxiety-related symptoms.

The stories in the book do not include this matter, because at the time of writing I did not realise it could be important. I had to wait for 24 hours before my delivery was induced. Recently I was reminded, by a friend I had not seen since Ellen was born, that I talked a lot about the anguish of waiting for the delivery. Several of the women in my investigation show distress in recalling the wait. One woman, however, was positive – she spent more than 24 hours at the ward, together with the staff, prior to the induction.

Further studies must be done on this question. In the meantime my advice is to make it routine to deliver the baby within hours of the diagnosis of fetal death. Women who themselves suggest waiting a while should be supported – but it is probably important to protect these women from meeting people who do not know about the death of the child. Such people may say something 'positive' about the future parenthood if they do not know what has happened.

My study indicates that women are less psychologically harmed from a stillbirth today than 30 years ago. One reason may be that before the introduction of prostaglandins and oxytocin to induce labour, women had to keep their dead child for weeks in the womb. This was a major psychological trauma, in addition to that of the stillbirth itself.

Afterwards

For the parents to have the opportunity, at the hospital, to commence the process of grieving for their child it is important that they can feel both independent and secure. It should be a matter of course that they may share a room on the ward. Enabling parents before, during and for a long time after the birth to meet the same midwife and doctor is probably especially advantageous. The midwife or doctor who assists at the delivery is often an important person. She or he may be freed from other duties to concentrate on these parents. The midwife may maintain contact with the parents even after the birth, thus requiring time to be set aside for her own consultations. It is desirable that there is a consistent strategy amongst the different members of staff with whom the parents come into contact. There should also be routines laid down which function during holidays and weekends.

During a crisis it is difficult to perceive and understand information. Explanations given to parents by the staff need to be repeated several times. What is said should be honest and sincere, and should not vary too much from staff member to staff member. Gynaecologists, paediatricians, midwives, medical social workers and psychologists can together develop a programme for postnatal care and from case to case decide who are most suitable members of staff to talk to the parents during and after their time at the hospital.

'An express train went through our home, a ball started rolling at great speed. There was a considerable distance between my husband and myself.' (Letter from Maria)

Grieving for a stillborn baby, or after a neonatal death, can continue for a long time. Grief can be more complicated when the baby is stillborn than when the baby is born alive but dies later. The parents have not even had the opportunity of holding their living baby in their arms.

If the baby is born deformed it can lead to the parents

brooding over what is wrong with them when they cannot have a normal baby. They grieve even for the healthy baby which they did not have.

'We had arranged flowers and wreaths with which we adorned the coffin. It looked so nice.' (Birgitta in 'Daring to try again')

If a funeral is held, it is very important that it is performed in accordance with the wishes of the parents, in order to make it a positive experience. It is a moment for reflection which gives the parents the chance to think about their future without the child they have just lost. If relatives and friends are present at the funeral then the child becomes 'visible' for more people, making it more difficult to forget or deny the baby's existence. At a grave the parents can tend the memory of the baby who died.

Daring to try again

Expecting a new baby brings back the pain of the memory of the dead baby.

'During the first half of the pregnancy I was psychologically unpregnant. I felt panic-stricken before going to the maternity clinic again, to sit there pregnant and to describe what had happened the previous time.' (Karin in 'Our Mårten')

It is important that the parents' anxiety is taken seriously. Extra checks are justifiable even if the pregnancy seems to be physically normal. To make light of their anxiety with comforting words, to tell them that this time everything will certainly go well, can have the opposite effect. How can one dare to believe that it will turn out well when things went so badly last time?

My investigation shows that a subsequent child improves the mother's self-esteem. Clearly, to have a new live child is important for most, if not all, women. We have little scientific evidence to support any advice about the timing of a new child. Probably we should not give any advice, or have any preconceptions on what is best. The parents' own intuitive feeling should guide us.

Knowledge and sympathy

'As a midwife, I wish that we would talk more about grief and reactions to crises.' (Meta in 'Be close, listen and be there...')

The care given to parents who have lost their baby can contribute to a fruitful process of grieving; it can however also make the reactions to grief more severe. Apart from the particular needs of parents of stillborn babies or babies who have suffered a neonatal death, the understanding of grief and care during crises is the basis of providing the correct form of support. On a labour ward we have the opportunity of sharing with the parents the incredible experience when a new person is born. The wish to assist on tragic occasions is probably not what makes someone choose to work on a maternity unit. Even so such occasions occur, fortunately rarely, but they are a reality at every unit.

Since, in many countries, fewer than one baby in a hundred dies at birth it is difficult for one person to acquire sufficient experience if he or she is not especially asked to attend deliveries of stillborn babies. In order to amass the common experience at a unit it is probably best that a group, consisting of a doctor, a midwife, a social worker, a psychologist and a hospital chaplain, continually assess how parents are given support. An important task for such a group is to create an environment where the staff can support one another at work.

'Even the distressing part of my work has enriched my life and developed me as a person. I feel a greater humility in life.'
(Meta in 'Be close, listen and be there...')

With knowledge and sympathy it is possible for a member of staff to give parents bereaved by a stillborn baby or a neonatal death, a memory which is worth cherishing. Such carers can look forward to meeting extremely grateful 'patients' at postnatal visits which take place much later. Instead of being something which one, as a staff member, would prefer to avoid, something frustrating, contact with parents who have lost their baby can be rewarding in many ways and be a part of the job, providing great satisfaction.

So, my own experience, the interviews in this book, my research and other studies can be summarized to the guidelines below. Some of this advice is firm – parents should see their baby for as long as they wish, and concrete reminders of the child should be collected. In other instances, as discussed above, future studies may alter our knowledge of what is optimal. Any guideline should be cautiously applied in practice – we must always listen to the needs of each individual mother and father.

Clinical guidelines

- Create a calm atmosphere in which the parents are able to spend as much time with their stillborn baby as they wish.

- Take a good photograph of the baby as soon as possible after the delivery.

- Secure tokens of remembrance such as a handprint, a footprint and a lock of hair from the baby.

- Induce labour as soon as possible after the diagnosis of death in utero – wait only when the mother takes an initiative or when it is necessary for practical reasons.

- Give the mother and father information and emotional support during the period between the confirmation of the child's death and the induction of labour.

- Be sensitive to any need for extra support for single women.

- Do not recommend a time limit for a new pregnancy after the stillbirth if there is no medical indication for it.

- Intensify the medical investigation to find out why the baby died.

- See the mother, or both parents, six months or so after the delivery. Such a visit will probably be rewarding for both you and the parents.

Afterword

To understand better how healthcare professionals can support women experiencing a stillbirth, I decided to initiate a survey. We used an anonymous questionnaire to collect data from 636 women who had given birth in Sweden in 1991. Of these women, 322 had given birth to live babies, and 314 had had babies which were stillborn. The investigation was nationwide, enabling us to study the variations in care around Sweden. We used population-based registers available in Sweden, to avoid problems with selection. To examine the long-term effects of different kinds of care, we assessed the women's anxiety-related symptoms at the time of follow-up, that is, three years after the delivery. You can find the results in the international medical literature (please see the reference list), and they are also included in my Doctoral Thesis.

A small increase in anxiety-related symptoms

The mean rating on the anxiety scale showed only a small difference between the women who had a stillborn baby and those who had a live one, and the median was identical among the groups. Women having been delivered of a stillborn child in Sweden in 1991 have, on average, only a small increase in the risk of anxiety-related symptoms. The increase in anxiety was seen in particular for single women, and among those in lower socio-economic groups.

Improved relationships

Our results indicate that stillbirth does not increase the risk of divorce. We found no differences in the estimated frequency of divorce or separation between the women who had a stillborn baby and those who gave birth to a live child. In both groups, 8 percent had separated from the child's father during the first three years after the delivery. For some women a stillbirth may result in a better relationship with the child's father. The women who had lost their baby reported more often than the controls that their relationship with the baby's father had improved after the stillbirth. Women whose children died in the womb gave a higher rating to satisfaction with their home and family situation. The results were the opposite, however, for single women. Single women having experienced stillbirth had a lower rating than single women with a live birth.

Lower self-esteem

Women who had lost a child had lower self-esteem than women who gave birth to a live baby. Twenty-five women (8%) who had lost their baby were not satisfied at all with their self-esteem, compared to 7 (2%) who had given birth to a live baby. Concerning their perception of their relationships outside the home, this variable was also reported by 8 percent of the women who had experienced a stillbirth and 2 percent of the women with a live birth. The figure was higher for women in the stillbirth group who had not subsequently given birth to a live child: 7 percent for stillbirth with a subsequent child and 12 percent for stillbirth without a new baby. The results indicate that a new baby may repair the impaired satisfaction to some extent. In our study, 140 women (45%) became pregnant within 6months of the stillbirth. Within 3 months, 69 (22%) of the women had become pregnant again and, within 1 year, 225 (75%) of the women.

The staff gave good support

More than 90 percent of the women felt that the attending staff showed respect for their stillborn baby and around 80 percent thought that the staff exhibited tenderness to the baby. The women's experience of support by the staff during labour and their perceptions of the staff's attitude to their baby was the same among the women who had stillborn babies and those who had live babies. These are high marks for members of staff who come into contact with the parents.

The time when the delivery of a stillborn child was regarded as a 'non-event' is over in Sweden. Today stillborns are treated as what they are – children. About 70 percent of the women with a stillborn baby thought that the hospital care routines were good and more than half of the women even felt that the delivery was a fine memory. At the same time nearly 40 percent had negative experiences. They reported that they were saddened, hurt, or angered by what some members of the staff had said or done.

Women who did not see their baby

Few women in 1991 did not see their stillborn baby. Thus, it is difficult, if not impossible, to study the effect of not seeing a child. In the study 14 women (4%) did not see their baby at all. In the questionnaire, six of them said they wished that they had seen their child. Four women were doubtful as to whether they ought to have seen the baby or not and 4 were still satisfied with having abstained.

It is possible that, for a small group of women, a 'real-life' confrontation with their stillborn baby would not be beneficial to their future wellbeing. By extrapolation from our survey figures, the number of such women would amount to 1 percent (4/314) – if the 4 women who did not see their baby and did not regret it at follow-up are counted.

Three women who never saw their baby stated that the staff had tried to persuade them to do so in an overly aggressive manner. None of the 300 women in the study who saw their baby – some of whom were persuaded to do so – regretted the event.

Together with her baby as long as she wishes

Women who were not able to be with their stillborn baby as long as they wished had a higher prevalence of anxiety-related symptoms than other women. If a mother does not see her stillborn child for as long as she wants to after the delivery she may suffer long-term psychological complications. When we instead measured the absolute time spent with the child, we found no certain correlation. 'As long as one wishes' is highly subjective; 10 minutes might be sufficient time for one woman, while 5 hours may be much too short a time for another. Some may need days, for example, by taking the baby home.

Memories of the baby

Our study demonstrates clearly the importance of preserving concrete reminders of the child. Women who have these have a reduced risk of long-term psychological complications. Examples of tokens are a satisfactory photograph, hand and footprints, a lock of hair, and an ultrasound image. More than one third of the women wished that they had more reminders of their child.

Ninety-four percent of the women had a photo of their stillborn baby. Nearly 50 of them (16%) were not satisfied with the picture. Sources of dissatisfaction include the arrangement, and the presence of postmortal changes that could have been avoided if the portrait was taken directly after the delivery.

The period between the diagnosis and induction

A clear correlation was found between the induction of labour more than 24 hours after the diagnosis of intrauterine fetal death and symptoms over the 90th percentile on the anxiety scale. We found a fivefold increase in risk of severe anxiety-related symptoms when the delivery was postponed more than 24 hours, and nearly a twofold increase for more than 6 hours. At the time of the study, many care providers routinely advised parents to go home after being informed that their baby was dead. The women were scheduled for induction of labour 1 or 2 days later. The present study highlights the need to investigate how women experience the time between the verification of the death of the baby and the induction of labour. We lack data in this respect.

Importance of knowing the cause of the stillbirth

Nearly all of the women in the study stated that it was important to know why their baby had died. Less than one third of the women had been given a definite explanation of the stillbirth, and over one third reported that they had not been given any explanation at all. Yet, using a comprehensive protocol, only in 12 percent of the intrauterine fatalities could no possible cause of death be ascertained (Ahlenius et al, 1995).

Articles from Doctoral Thesis

Rådestad I. Att föda ett dött barn - Vården vid förlossningen och kvinnans situation tre år efter barnets död (Doctoral Thesis). Stockholm: Karolinska Institute; 1998.

Rådestad I, Steineck G, Nordin C, Sjögren B. Psychological complications after stillbirth – Influence of memories and immediate management: Population based study. BMJ 1996;312:1505-1508.

Rådestad I, Sjögren B, Nordin C, Steineck G. Stillbirth is no longer managed as a non-event – A nationwide study. Birth Issues in Perinatal Care 1996;23:209-215.

Rådestad I, Nordin C, Steineck G, Sjögren B. Stillbirth and maternal wellbeing – Population based survey. Acta Obstet Gynecol Scand 1997;76:849-855.

Rådestad I, Nordin C, Steineck G, Sjögren B. Women's memories and views of pregnancy and delivery after stillbirth. Midwifery 1998;14:111-117.

Rådestad I, Otterblad-Olausson P, Steineck G. Aspects of measuring errors and non-responses in a nationwide study of stillbirth. Acta Obst Gyn Scand 1999 (at press).

Support Groups

Child Bereavement Trust
Brindley House
4 Burkes Road
Beaconsfield
Bucks. HP9 1TP
Tel: 01494 678088
Fax: 01494 678765

Child Death Helpline
Bereavement Services
Department
Great Ormond Street Hospital
for Children NHS Trust
London WC1N 3JH
Tel: 0171 813 8550/1
Fax: 0171 813 8516
HELPLINE: 0800 282986

The Compassionate Friends
53 North Street
Bristol
BS3 1EN
Tel: 0117 966 5202
Fax: 0117 966 5202
HELPLINE: 0117 953 9639

Cruse – Bereavement Care
Cruse House
126 Sheen Road
Richmond
Surrey TW9 1UR
(Send SAE for free booklet)
Tel: 0181 940 4818
Fax: 0181 940 7638
HELPLINE: 0181 332 7227

Miscarriage Association
c/o Clayton Hospital
Northgate
Wakefield
West Yorkshire WF1 3JS
Tel: 01924 200799
Fax: 01924 298834

Perinatal Bereavement Unit
The Tavistock Clinic
120 Belsize Lane
London NW3 5BA
Tel: 0171 435 7111
Fax: 0171 431 8978

Stillbirth and Neonatal Death Society
(SANDS)
28 Portland Place
London W1N 4DE
Tel: 0171 436 7940
Fax: 0171 436 3715
HELPLINE: 0171 436 3715